Pediatric Prevention

Editor

HENRY S. ROANE

PEDIATRIC CLINICS
OF NORTH AMERICA

www.pediatric.theclinics.com

Consulting Editor
BONITA F. STANTON

June 2020 • Volume 67 • Number 3

ELSEVIER

1600 John F. Kennedy Boulevard • Suite 1800 • Philadelphia, Pennsylvania, 19103-2899

http://www.theclinics.com

THE PEDIATRIC CLINICS OF NORTH AMERICA Volume 67, Number 3
June 2020 ISSN 0031-3955, ISBN-13: 978-0-323-73384-7

Editor: Kerry Holland
Developmental Editor: Casey Potter

The Pediatric Clinics of North America (ISSN 0031-3955) is published bimonthly by Elsevier Inc., 360 Park Avenue South, New York, NY 10010-1710. Months of issue are February, April, June, August, October, and December. Periodicals postage paid at New York, NY and additional mailing offices. Subscription prices are $240.00 per year (US individuals), $695.00 per year (US institutions), $315.00 per year (Canadian individuals), $924.00 per year (Canadian institutions), $362.00 per year (international individuals), $924.00 per year (international institutions), $100.00 per year (US students and residents), $100.00 per year (Canadian students and residents), and $165.00 per year (international residents and students). To receive students/resident rare, orders must be accompanied by name of affiliated institution, date of term, and the signature of program/residency coordinator on institution letterhead. Orders will be billed at individual rate until proof of status is received. Foreign air speed delivery is included in all *Clinics* subscription prices. All prices are subject to change without notice. **POSTMASTER:** Send address changes to *The Pediatric Clinics of North America*, Elsevier Health Sciences Division, Subscription Customer Service, 3251 Riverport Lane, Maryland Heights, MO 63043. **Customer Service: 1-800-654-2452 (US and Canada). From outside of the US and Canada: 1-314-447-8871. Fax: 1-314-447-8029. For print support, E-mail: JournalsCustomerService-usa@elsevier.com. For online support, E-mail: JournalsOnlineSupport-usa@elsevier.com.**

Reprints. For copies of 100 or more, of articles in this publication, please contact the Commercial Reprints Department, Elsevier Inc., 360 Park Avenue South, New York, NY 10010-1710. Tel.: 212-633-3874; Fax: 212-633-3820; E-mail: reprints@elsevier.com.

The Pediatric Clinics of North America is also published in Spanish by McGraw-Hill Inter-americana Editores S.A., Mexico City, Mexico; in Portuguese by Riechmann and Affonso Editores, Rua Comandante Coelho 1085, CEP 21250, Rio de Janeiro, Brazil; and in Greek by Althayia SA, Athens, Greece.

The Pediatric Clinics of North America is covered in *MEDLINE/PubMed (Index Medicus), Excerpta Medica, Current Contents, Current Contents/Clinical Medicine, Science Citation Index, ASCA, ISI/BIOMED,* and *BIOSIS.*

PROGRAM OBJECTIVE

The goal of the *Pediatric Clinics of North America* is to keep practicing physicians and residents up to date with current clinical practice in pediatrics by providing timely articles reviewing the state-of-the-art in patient care.

TARGET AUDIENCE

All practicing pediatricians, physicians and healthcare professionals who provide patient care to pediatric patients.

LEARNING OBJECTIVES

Upon completion of this activity, participants will be able to:
1. Review pediatric behavioral concerns and mitigating risks for developing behavioral disorders.
2. Discuss pediatric health and wellness topics such as academic behavior, oral care, weight management, substance use disorders and safety skills.
3. Recognize secondary and tertiary prevention of autism spectrum disorder, feeding disorders, severe behavior problems associated with intellectual and developmental disabilities, tic disorders, and sleep disorders.

ACCREDITATIONS

Physician Credit

The Elsevier Office of Continuing Medical Education (EOCME) is accredited by the Accreditation Council for Continuing Medical Education (ACCME) to provide continuing medical education for physicians.

The EOCME designates this journal-based activity for a maximum of 13 *AMA PRA Category 1 Credit*(s)™. Physicians should claim only the credit commensurate with the extent of their participation in the activity.

All other healthcare professionals requesting continuing education credit for this this journal-based activity will be issued a certificate of participation.

ABP Maintenance of Certification Credit

Successful completion of this CME activity, which includes participation in the activity and individual assessment of and feedback to the learner, enables the learner to earn up to 13 MOC points in the American Board of Pediatrics' (ABP) Maintenance of Certification (MOC) program. It is the CME activity provider's responsibility to submit learner completion information to ACCME for the purpose of granting ABP MOC credit.

DISCLOSURE OF CONFLICTS OF INTEREST

The EOCME assesses conflict of interest with its instructors, faculty, planners, and other individuals who are in a position to control the content of CME activities. All relevant conflicts of interest that are identified are thoroughly vetted by EOCME for fair balance, scientific objectivity, and patient care recommendations. EOCME is committed to providing its learners with CME activities that promote improvements or quality in healthcare and not a specific proprietary business or a commercial interest.

The planning committee, staff, authors and editors listed below have identified no financial relationships or relationships to products or devices they or their spouse/life partner have with commercial interest related to the content of this CME activity:
Keith D. Allen, PhD; Ashley S. Andersen, MS, BCBA; Iram J. Ashraf, MD; Emily L. Baxter, MA, BCBA; Jordan Belisle, PhD; Samantha Bergmann, PhD; Ann S. Botash, MD; Jodi Coon, MS; Jaime G. Crowley, PhD, BCBA-D; Mark R. Dixon, PhD; Laura Fisher; Patrick C. Friman, PhD; J. Logan Gibson, BS; Louis P. Hagopian, PhD, BCBA-D; Sarah D. Haney, MA, BCBA; Kerry Holland; Vivian F. Ibañez, PhD, BCBA-D; Marilu Kelly, MSN, RN, CNE, CHCP; Tiffany Kodak, PhD; Sara Kupzyk, PhD; Patricia F. Kurtz, PhD; Mauro Leoni, PhD; Odessa Luna, PhD; Brian K. Martens, PhD; Rajkumar Mayakrishnann; Raymond G. Miltenberger, PhD, BCBA-D; Christopher P. Morley, PhD; Matthew P. Normand, PhD; Alicia R. Pekarsky, MD; Kathryn M. Peterson, PhD, BCBA-D; Cathleen C. Piazza, PhD, BCBA-D; JoAnne E. Race, MS; John T. Rapp, PhD; Alicia C. Reyes, MPH; Henry S. Roane, PhD; Sindy Sanchez, PhD, BCBA-D; Connie J. Schnoes, PhD; Jordan T. Stiede, BA; Diego Valbuena, PhD, BCBA-D.

The planning committee, staff, authors and editors listed below have identified financial relationships or relationships to products or devices they or their spouse/life partner have with commercial interest related to the content of this CME activity:
Douglas W. Woods, PhD: receives royalties from Oxford University Press, Springer Nature Switzerland AG, and Guilford Press.

UNAPPROVED/OFF-LABEL USE DISCLOSURE

The EOCME requires CME faculty to disclose to the participants:

1. When products or procedures being discussed are off-label, unlabelled, experimental, and/or investigational (not US Food and Drug Administration [FDA] approved); and
2. Any limitations on the information presented, such as data that are preliminary or that represent ongoing research, interim analyses, and/or unsupported opinions. Faculty may discuss information about pharmaceutical agents that is outside of FDA-approved labelling. This information is intended solely for CME and is not intended to promote off-label use of these medications. If you have any questions, contact the medical affairs department of the manufacturer for the most recent prescribing information.

TO ENROLL

To enroll in the *Pediatric Clinics of North America* Continuing Medical Education program, call customer service at 1-800-654-2452 or sign up online at http://www.theclinics.com/home/cme. The CME program is available to subscribers for an additional annual fee of USD 300.00.

METHOD OF PARTICIPATION

In order to claim credit, participants must complete the following:

1. Complete enrolment as indicated above.
2. Read the activity.
3. Complete the CME Test and Evaluation. Participants must achieve a score of 70% on the test. All CME Tests and Evaluations must be completed online.

In order to claim MOC points, participants must complete the following:

1. Complete steps listed above for claiming CME credit
2. Provide your specialty board ID#, birth date (MM/DD), and attestation.
3. Online MOC submission is only available for the American Board of pediatrics' (ABP) Maintenance of Certification (MOC) program

CME INQUIRIES/SPECIAL NEEDS

For all CME inquiries or special needs, please contact elsevierCME@elsevier.com.

Contributors

CONSULTING EDITOR

BONITA F. STANTON, MD
Founding Dean, Hackensack Meridian School of Medicine at Seton Hall University, President, Academic Enterprise, Hackensack Meridian Health Robert C. and Laura C. Garrett Endowed Chair for the School of Medicine, Professor of Pediatrics, Nutley, New Jersey, USA

EDITOR

HENRY S. ROANE, PhD
The G.S. Liptak Professor of Child Development, Chief, Division of Development, Behavior and Genetics, Professor, Departments of Pediatrics and Psychiatry, SUNY Upstate Medical University, Syracuse, New York, USA

AUTHORS

KEITH D. ALLEN, PhD
Professor, Psychology, Munroe-Meyer Institute for Genetics and Rehabilitation, University of Nebraska Medical Center, Omaha, Nebraska, USA

ASHLEY S. ANDERSEN, MS, BCBA
Munroe-Meyer Institute, University of Nebraska Medical Center, Omaha, Nebraska, USA

IRAM J. ASHRAF, MD
Fellow, Child Abuse Pediatrics, Department of Pediatrics, SUNY Upstate Medical University, Upstate Golisano Children's Hospital, Syracuse, New York, USA

EMILY L. BAXTER, MA
Department of Psychology, Syracuse University, Syracuse, New York, USA

JORDAN BELISLE, PhD
Assistant Professor, Applied Behavior Analysis, Psychology Department, Missouri State University, Springfield, Missouri, USA

SAMANTHA BERGMANN, PhD, BCBA-D
Assistant Professor, Department of Behavior Analysis, University of North Texas, Denton, Texas, USA

ANN S. BOTASH, MD
SUNY Distinguished Teaching Professor, Department of Pediatrics, SUNY Upstate Medical University, Upstate Golisano Children's Hospital, Syracuse, New York, USA

JODI COON, MS, BCBA
APMRT, Auburn University, Auburn, Alabama, USA

JAIME G. CROWLEY, PhD, BCBA-D
May Institute, Randolph, Massachusetts, USA

MARK R. DIXON, PhD
Department of Disability and Human Development, University of Illinois at Chicago, Chicago, Illinois, USA

PATRICK C. FRIMAN, PhD
Vice President, Center for Behavioral Health, Boys Town, Nebraska, USA

JOSHUA LOGAN GIBSON, BS
Graduate Student, Department of Psychology, University of the Pacific, Stockton, California, USA

LOUIS P. HAGOPIAN, PhD, BCBA-D
Professor, Department of Psychiatry and Behavioral Sciences, Johns Hopkins School of Medicine, Program Director, Neurobehavioral Unit, Kennedy Krieger Institute, Baltimore, Maryland, USA

SARAH D. HANEY, PhD, BCBA
Munroe-Meyer Institute, University of Nebraska Medical Center, Omaha, Nebraska, USA

VIVIAN F. IBAÑEZ, PhD, BCBA-D
Children's Specialized Hospital and Rutgers University, Somerset, New Jersey, USA

TIFFANY KODAK, PhD, BCBA-D
Associate Professor, Department of Psychology, Marquette University, Milwaukee, Wisconsin, USA

SARA KUPZYK, PhD
Assistant Professor, Psychology, University of Nebraska, Omaha, Nebraska, USA

PATRICIA F. KURTZ, PhD
Director, Neurobehavioral Outpatient Services, Neurobehavioral Unit, Kennedy Krieger Institute, Associate Professor, Department of Psychiatry and Behavioral Sciences, Johns Hopkins School of Medicine, Baltimore, Maryland, USA

MAURO LEONI, PhD
Consultant Psychologist and Behavior Analyst, Department of Disabilities, Fondazione Istituto Ospedaliero di Sospiro Onlus, Sospiro (CR), Italy; Professor, Freud University of Milan, Milan, Italy

ODESSA LUNA, PhD, BCBA
Assistant Professor of Applied Behavior Analysis, Community Psychology, Saint Cloud, Minnesota, USA

BRIAN K. MARTENS, PhD
Department of Psychology, Syracuse University, Syracuse, New York, USA

RAYMOND G. MILTENBERGER, PhD, BCBA-D
Professor, Department of Child and Family Studies, University of South Florida, Tampa, Florida, USA

CHRISTOPHER P. MORLEY, PhD
Associate Professor and Chair, Department of Public Health and Preventive Medicine, Associate Professor and Vice Chair for Research, Department of Family Medicine,

Associate Professor, Department of Psychiatry and Behavioral Sciences, Upstate Medical University, Syracuse, New York, USA

MATTHEW P. NORMAND, PhD
Professor, Department of Psychology, University of the Pacific, Stockton, California, USA

ALICIA R. PEKARSKY, MD
Associate Professor, Department of Pediatrics, SUNY Upstate Medical University, Upstate Golisano Children's Hospital, Syracuse, New York, USA

KATHRYN M. PETERSON, PhD, BCBA-D
Children's Specialized Hospital and Rutgers University, Somerset, New Jersey, USA

CATHLEEN C. PIAZZA, PhD, BCBA-D
Rutgers University Graduate School of Applied and Professional Psychology and Children's Specialized Hospital, Somerset, New Jersey, USA

JOANNE E. RACE, MS
Instructor, Department of Pediatrics, SUNY Upstate Medical University, Upstate Golisano Children's Hospital, Syracuse, New York, USA

JOHN T. RAPP, PhD, BCBA-D
Alumni Professor, Director of the Applied Behavior Analysis Program, Project Director, APMRT, Auburn University, Auburn, Alabama, USA

ALICIA C. REYES, MPH
Medical Student (MS1), MPH Program Alum, Upstate Medical University, College of Medicine, Syracuse, New York, USA

SINDY SANCHEZ, PhD, BCBA-D
Co-Owner, Comprehensive Behavioral Consulting, Tampa, Florida, USA

CONNIE J. SCHNOES, PhD
Director, National Behavioral Health Dissemination, Center for Behavioral Health, Boys Town, Nebraska, USA

JORDAN T. STIEDE, BA
Clinical Psychology PhD Student, Psychology Department, Marquette University, Milwaukee, Wisconsin, USA

DIEGO VALBUENA, PhD, BCBA-D
Co-Owner, Comprehensive Behavioral Consulting, Tampa, Florida, USA

DOUGLAS W. WOODS, PhD
Vice Provost for Graduate and Professional Studies and Dean of the Graduate School, Professor of Psychology, Marquette University, Milwaukee, Wisconsin, USA

Contents

As members of state-funded team to monitor psychotropic medication use and examine cost-effective methods for behavioral treatment in foster care, the authors review behavioral studies on interventions for foster youth who engage in challenging behavior. Four behavioral technologies—preference assessments, teaching procedures, functional behavioral assessment and intervention, and parent training—are discussed. Four case studies and behavioral data for foster youth treated using these technologies are provided. Finally, pediatric providers are encouraged to recommend a practitioner with specialized training in behavior analysis to foster parents if a child displays disruptive behavior.

Applied behavior analysis has the most empirical support as intervention for pediatric feeding disorders, when a child does not eat or drink a sufficient quantity or variety of food to maintain proper nutrition. Interdisciplinary collaboration is crucial for diagnosis, referral, and management of pediatric feeding disorders because the etiology is complex and multifactorial. Thus, our aim is to provide information about how to recognize a feeding disorder, to delineate the environmental variables implicated in the etiology and maintenance of feeding disorders, and to provide recommendations for prevention and intervention for feeding disorders based on the applied-behavior analytic literature.

Many children in the United States are performing below basic standards in reading, mathematics, and writing. Children at risk for academic problems often have comorbid classroom behavior problems and/or are diagnosed with high-incidence disabilities. Early intervention to prevent academic problems is a key goal of school-wide response-to-intervention models. The goal of school-based instructional intervention is to increase children's strength of responding so basic academic skills can be combined to solve more complex tasks. Parents and caregivers can support

individuals and can be a costly disorder across one's lifetime. Because of the prevalence, costs, and range of behavioral needs, early intervention is vital to teach skills across a variety of domains and prevent the development or exacerbation of behavioral deficits and excesses. Interventions based on applied behavior analysis have the most empirical support; several strategies to teach social skills, communication, and adaptive skills are discussed.

Obesity has become a public health crisis associated with serious health problems. It is a problem that is, by and large, remarkably simple: you gain weight as a result of consuming more calories than you burn. Applied behavior analysis and behavior therapy have produced a range of methods and technologies well-suited to address the problems of overeating and physical inactivity. These methods and technologies, and the conceptual foundations underpinning them, are the focus of this article.

It is not clear whether the development of tics can be prevented. Contextual variables can impact tic expression; therefore, shifting attention to behaviors that reduce tics is an important part of decreasing tic severity. Several medications are effective in reducing tic severity, but side effects restrict their use. Behavioral treatment is the gold standard psychotherapy intervention for tic disorders, with Comprehensive Behavioral Intervention for Tics being the most well-supported nonpharmacological treatment. Although children may be unable to prevent the development of tics, they can still use several strategies to reduce tic severity and impairment.

This article addresses the essential role of sleep in the medical, emotional, behavioral, and cognitive health of children. Sleep disorders common among children are defined along with the most common sleep concerns reported by caregivers. Prevention and intervention strategies are described.

Serious threats to child safety are infrequent and unpredictable but can lead to serious injury and death. To stay safe, children must identify and avoid contact with a safety threat, escape from it, and report it to an adult so the adult can remove the threat. Research shows that active learning approaches are effective for teaching children to engage in these safety skills. Passive learning approaches are not effective. Active learning approaches require children to practice the skills in the presence of simulated

threats with feedback to reinforce correct responses and promote generalization of skills to the natural environment.

Prevention amounts to stopping a disease from occurring, either through
avoidance of risk factors, or through prophylactic measures, such as
vaccination, use of barrier methods during sexual encounters, and so
forth. However, as one delves into the topic of prevention, it becomes
apparent that there are multiple points for intervention into a disease,
that the stage of disease matters as to what preventive actions are appropriate, the type of disease, and even the overlapping concepts of disease
versus illness.

Behavior and substance use addictions are increasingly prevalent in children with increased risk for substance abuse and mental health diagnoses
in adulthood. This article proposes a comprehensive model of addiction to
inform research on the prevention and treatment of childhood addiction,
emphasizing skills training, mindfulness training, and broader treatment
strategies consistent with acceptance and commitment therapy.

PEDIATRIC CLINICS OF NORTH AMERICA

SERIES OF RELATED INTEREST

Clinics in Perinatology
http://www.perinatology.theclinics.com/
Advances in Pediatrics
http://www.advancesinpediatrics.com/

THE CLINICS ARE AVAILABLE ONLINE!
Access your subscription at:
www.theclinics.com

Foreword

Prevention: An Essential Part of Pediatrics

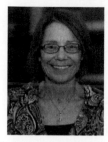

Bonita F. Stanton, MD
Consulting Editor

Life expectancy in the United States relative to our peer nations has suffered greatly over the past several decades. In the 1950s, the United States enjoyed a life expectancy among the top 5 nations in the world.[1] Currently, US life expectancy is now among the bottom half of the Organization for Economic Co-operation and Development nations.[2]

Prevention and life expectancy are highly correlated. As preventive efforts increase, so too does life expectancy. Prevention is critical at all stages of life. No where is prevention more effective—and more essential—than during infancy and childhood. Prevention efforts during this timeframe greatly increase not only the chances of a healthy infancy and childhood but also the chances of a far healthier and longer life overall. The importance of early prevention efforts is not controversial and is not contested. Indeed, greater attention to both prevention efforts throughout the lifespan and particularly those in infancy and childhood is needed to maximize both the duration and the quality of life in the United States.[3]

This issue of *Pediatric Clinics of North America*, entitled "Pediatric Prevention," focuses on a range of prevention efforts that offers great promise when initiated during childhood. Several of the articles address broad issues of prevention ("Pediatric Prevention: General Prevention"), while most of the remaining articles focus on a wide range of critical areas, including feeding disorders, academic performance, oral hygiene, and sleep dysfunction. Other articles describe approaches to identifying parenting problems that can be identified and modified to prevent subsequent child disorders, such as preventing child abuse and identifying early on behaviors that left undiagnosed and untreated can result in significant behavioral disorders. Several articles identify conditions such as autism, which if identified and treated early can greatly mitigate the course of the disorder.

Pediatr Clin N Am 67 (2020) xv–xvi
https://doi.org/10.1016/j.pcl.2020.03.003
0031-3955/20/© 2020 Published by Elsevier Inc.

pediatric.theclinics.com

This is an important issue for all pediatricians and other child health care professionals. Each of the articles addresses issues of great importance and opportunity for amelioration during childhood with the probability of either or both a longer and healthier adulthood.

Bonita F. Stanton, MD
Hackensack Meridian School of Medicine at Seton Hall University
340 Kingsland Street, Building 123
Nutley, NJ 07110, USA

E-mail address:
bonita.stanton@shu.edu

REFERENCES

1. OECD Factbook 2007: economic, environmental and social statistics. Available at: http://www.oecd.org. Accessed April 6, 2020.
2. OECD. Life expectancy at birth. Available at: https://data.oecd.org/healthstat/life-expectancy-at-birth.htm. Accessed April 6, 2020.
3. Maciosek MV, Coffield AB, Flottemesch TJ, et al. Greater use of preventive services in US health care could save lives at little or no cost. Health Aff (Millwood) 2010;29(9):1656–60.

Preface

Pediatric Prevention

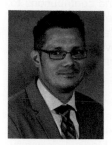

Henry S. Roane, PhD
Editor

At the time of this writing, we are dealing with the COVID-19 pandemic. Our society is constantly being reminded of preventative procedures against exposure to this virus: hand washing, covering your cough, social distancing. These types of prevention behavior represent primary prevention in that their intent is to prevent spread of a disease to an unaffected population (see Morley and Reyes, this issue), and it is primary prevention that readers likely have the greatest familiarity with. However, preventative care may also involve the application of empirically derived practices to those precursor behaviors that might develop into a larger health concern by mitigating the risk of worsening outcomes. Such secondary and tertiary prevention is the focus of the current issue.

Within the context of pediatric behavioral concerns and remediating those factors that place a child at risk for developing behavioral concerns, prevention focuses not only on intervention early during a child's development (to prevent worsening) but also on decreasing the long-term sequela of the targeted concern. The articles presented in this issue address behaviorally based preventative measures that have a history of evidence-based care in pediatric populations. The content includes prevention of problematic behavior associated with foster care placement as well as the prevention of child abuse. Both are conditions that can give rise to a range of childhood behavior disorders. As well, there are condition-specific disorders for which there is well-established literature on secondary and tertiary prevention. These include the current topics of autism spectrum disorder, feeding disorders, severe behavior problems associated with intellectual and developmental disabilities, tic disorders, and sleep disorders. Finally, some of the content of the issue addresses broader health and wellness within pediatric populations. This includes contributions on academic behavior, oral care, weight management, and substance use disorders (eg, drug consumption, excessive video game play), as well as an article on teaching a range of safety skills (eg, gun safety, abduction prevention) to children.

Pediatr Clin N Am 67 (2020) xvii–xviii
https://doi.org/10.1016/j.pcl.2020.03.002
0031-3955/20/© 2020 Published by Elsevier Inc.

One common theme across these articles is their basis in the behavioral sciences, particularly applied behavior analysis (ABA), which is a clinical discipline wherein the general principles of learning and behavior are applied for the purpose of addressing socially relevant problems. One of the most notable features of ABA is its focus on direct observation and data collection to inform intervention decision making. The emphasis on data-based decision making is evident in each of the contributions to this issue. The goal of this issue is to address socially relevant behavioral problems common as referrals to pediatric practices and to make providers aware of the range of treatment options available to patients, as well as informing providers of evidence-based strategies for identifying precursors and preventing further worsening of behavior problems in children.

Henry S. Roane, PhD
Division of Development, Behavior and Genetics
Departments of Pediatrics and Psychiatry
SUNY Upstate Medical University
750 East Adams Street
Syracuse, NY 13210, USA

E-mail address:
roaneh@upstate.edu

Enhancing the Lives of Foster Youth with Behavioral Interventions

Odessa Luna, PhD, BCBA[a], John T. Rapp, PhD, BCBA-D[b],*,
Jodi Coon, MS, BCBA[b]

KEYWORDS

- Applied behavior analysis • Behavioral intervention • Disruptive behavior
- Foster care • Foster parent • Functional behavioral assessment • Parent training
- Problem behavior

KEY POINTS

- Foster youth may engage in challenging behavior that may result in multiple placements and the prescription of psychotropic medication.
- Practitioners in applied behavior analysis (board-certified behavior analysts [BCBAs]) are highly suited to assess and treat foster youth's disruptive behavior in homes and other residential settings.
- BCBAs design behavioral treatment by arranging the environment to increase appropriate foster youth behavior while reducing disruptive behavior.
- Foster parents are key agents of change for foster youth. BCBAs can teach parents how to promote pivotal skills and decrease maladaptive behavior in their homes for foster youth.
- Pediatric providers should direct parents whose foster children display problem behavior to a BCBA.

INTRODUCTION

In 2016, more than 400,000 children experienced parental or guardian abuse, neglect, or both.[1] Due to the severity of such experiences, state agencies often are required to place these children in a 24-hour substitute, foster care.[2] Compared with children outside of foster care, foster youth are more likely to engage in externalizing behaviors (inappropriate language, aggression, and noncompliance), which may give rise to practitioners diagnosing these children with emotional behavioral disorder.[3] Additionally, foster youth often lack important life skills[4] and are more likely that children who reside with their biological parents to receive psychotropic medication[5] to treat behavioral excesses. Once removed from their home, these abused and neglected youth

[a] Community Psychology, Education Building, 720 4th Avenue South, Saint Cloud, MN 56301, USA; [b] APMRT, Auburn University, 226 Thach, Auburn, AL 36849, USA
* Corresponding author.
E-mail address: jtr0014@auburn.edu

Pediatr Clin N Am 67 (2020) 437–449
https://doi.org/10.1016/j.pcl.2020.02.001
0031-3955/20/Published by Elsevier Inc.

enter placements with unfamiliar rules, expectations, and individuals. Furthermore, when foster children engage in disruptive behavior, a series of untoward events can ensue. One such negative event can include *placement disruption*, a term coined to describe a situation in which a foster child moves to another foster placement (other foster homes, group homes, residential facilities, and hospitals).[6]

During a placement disruption, children are likely to miss school, have limited access to their home community, and may develop further additional behavioral concerns.[7] Additionally, children who have been through the child welfare system are less likely to obtain a high school diploma or general equivalency degree,[8] more likely to be incarcerated before 21 years of age,[9] more likely to be pregnant as a teenager,[10] and more likely to be homeless as an adult.[11] Given these detrimental possibilities that foster youth may experience, in particular youth who experience placement disruption, it is imperative that pediatricians are aware that there is a science of behavior. This science, applied behavior analysis (ABA), is well suited to prevention solutions for this vulnerable population.

In part, ABA consists of the assessment and treatment of socially significant human behavior.[12] Key tenets of behavior analysis include the measurement of observable behaviors, frequent assessment, and individualized interventions targeted to increase appropriate behavior and decrease inappropriate behavior. Board-certified behavior analysts [BCBAs] (ie, practitioners in ABA) endorse a pragmatic philosophy of behavior. Specifically, by recognizing that the environment (other people) reinforces behavior throughout the life an individual,[13] BCBAs can design interventions that promote positive, social behaviors and decrease maladaptive, problematic behaviors. As such, BCBAs design assessments and interventions that target challenging behavior of foster youth without relying on psychotropic medication, restraint, or seclusion.

BEHAVIORAL TECHNOLOGIES FOR FOSTER CARE YOUTH

The Child and Family Services Improvement and Innovation Act (2011)[14] mandated that states develop systems to monitor psychotropic medication usage. Based on this legislation, the Deputy Director of the Alabama Department of Human Resources proposed the development of a behavioral health team, collectively known as the Alabama Psychiatric Medication Review Team (APMRT). The APMRT is composed of a board-certified child psychiatrist, a psychiatric nurse practitioner, a psychopharmacologist, and several BCBAs. One task of the APMRT is evaluating the extent to which behavioral interventions can be used as safer alternatives to psychotropic medication for managing problem behavior for children in Alabama foster care. As indicated by **Fig. 1**, the APMRT served 98 foster children who presented with a variety of behavioral challenges and their foster families from August 2017 to April 2019. The purpose of this article is to outline empirical studies that used behavioral technologies with foster youth. Case studies from the authors' work on the APMRT also are reviewed to illustrate the impact that empirically based behavioral assessment and intervention can have on the life of a foster child. Although the authors used numerous behavioral prevention strategies with each foster child, each case study illustrates a specific prevention tool used within a larger treatment package.

Preference Assessments

Broadly, preference assessments are empirically supported assessment tools that identify snacks, items, activities, and privileges a foster child may enjoy.[15] BCBAs can utilize the outcomes of a preference assessment in 3 different ways to prioritize the well-being of the foster child. First, preference assessments can be particularly

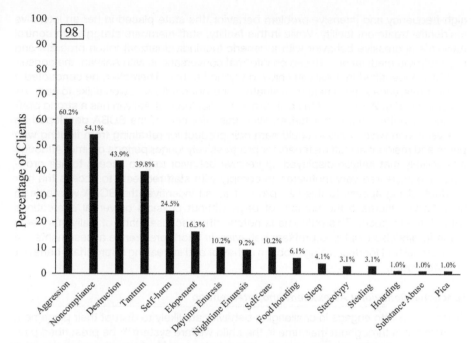

Fig. 1. An overall summary of the referring behavioral concerns for clients served by the APMRT. Since 2017, the authors have worked with approximately 98 children with a variety of behavioral concerns in foster homes, residential settings, and schools. Some children were referred for multiple problem behaviors.

helpful when foster youth are transitioning into a foster placement. For example, the outcomes may reveal a foster child loves a certain genre of music. Therefore, a child's treatment team could work together to ensure preferred music is available when the foster child arrives in the new home, potentially mitigating anxiety and fear associated with the new placement.[16]

Second, preference assessments can aid service providers in the selection of incentives a child may be motivated to earn for appropriate behaviors, such as completing household chores, self-care responsibilities, and academic tasks. For instance, a preference assessment may reveal that a child is highly motivated to gain access to electronic devices. The BCBA may recommend to the foster parent to allow 10 minutes of a preferred activity after completion of chores.

Third, preference assessments may provide key details that aid in the design of behavior reduction strategies. For instance, a foster child's preference assessment may indicate that she likes social interaction (eg, visiting with friends, talking to family, and playing board games). Based on such results, the BCBA and foster parent could prioritize goals, such as teaching the child appropriate social skills, making her less likely to display problematic behaviors, such as cursing, running away, hitting others, or shutting down. The following case description briefly illustrates how a preference assessment can inform the development of a behavioral intervention.

Case Study 1

An APMRT BCBA worked with Aaliyah, a 13-year-old girl diagnosed with major depressive disorder and attention-deficit/hyperactivity disorder (ADHD). Due to high-frequency and intensive problem behavior, the state placed in her an intensive residential treatment facility. While in this facility, staff members struggled to control Aaliyah's aggressive behavior with a generic (nonindividualized) token program and psychotropic medications. Based on informal conversations with Aaliyah, the consulting BCBA identified that Aaliyah enjoyed styling her hair. Thereafter, he conducted a formal preference assessment to evaluate hair products Aaliyah would like to earn. As indicated in **Fig. 2**, results of the assessment indicated that Aaliyah has a strong preference for butter cream moisturizer. With this information, the BCBA developed an intervention in which Aaliyah could earn hair product for refraining from fighting with peers and residential staff members for progressively longer periods of time. Although it is unlikely that Aaliyah displayed aggressive behavior to gain access to hair products, she appeared very motivated to comply with staff requests to access the hair product. Using access to this hair product as an incentive, the BCBA was able to help Aaliyah increase the number of days without physical or verbal altercations with staff and peers. This outcome is noteworthy because many of Aaliyah's peers in the facility also displayed problem behavior. In short, preference assessments are an essential tool for decreasing problem behavior and increasing appropriate behavior in foster youth.

Functional Behavioral Assessment and Intervention

Foster youth who engage in challenging behavior are likely to disrupt their placement multiple times throughout their time in the child welfare system[16]; be prescribed psychotropic medications to decrease disruptive behaviors,[17] which often have negative

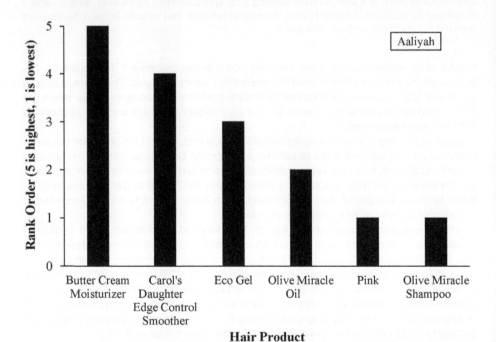

Fig. 2. Preference assessment results indicating that Aaliyah had a high preference for butter cream moisturizer when given the choice of 5 other hair products. This information aided the BCBA in developing an effective behavioral intervention to reduce Aaliyah's fighting behavior against staff members and peers in an intensive residential facility.

side effects[18,19]; or both. Given the detrimental effects of placement disruption and increased likelihood of a psychotropic medication prescription,[20] pediatricians should recommend and encourage the use of evidence-based behavioral assessment and intervention practices.[21]

One such evidence-based practice, a functional behavior assessment (FBA), is the process of identifying environmental variables that contribute to disruptive behaviors by foster children. This assessment process may encompass rating scales,[22] parent interviews,[23] observational data,[24] and deliberate manipulation of specific environmental variables (ie, functional analysis[25]). These assessments can help determine if disruptive behavior occurs to gain attention from others (parents, teachers, and peers), avoid or escape tasks (chores, homework, and social interactions), gain access to activities or items, or contact self-stimulating sensations.[26] As a simple example, an FBA may indicate that a foster child learned to a strike a foster sibling to gain access a sibling's toy. The consulting BCBA may, for example, develop an intervention that teaches the foster child to appropriately request the sibling's toy, exchange toys with the sibling, or both.

In general, research indicates that function-based interventions produce more clinically desirable outcomes than interventions unrelated to the function of the problem behavior.[27,28] Researchers used FBA tools to assess and then treat runaway behavior in foster youth.[27] Thereafter, they compared the outcomes to a matched-control sample. The FBAs revealed that many individuals in the treatment group ran away to (1) escape or avoid unpleasant environmental conditions of the foster placement (eg, activity restrictions and feeling alienated) and gain access to family members, friends, and significant others or (2) engage in drug or sexual activities. For individuals assessed with FBAs, BCBAs designed interventions specific to the function of running away. For example, if the foster youth ran away to see preferred people in their lives (biological family), the BCBA worked with service providers to schedule frequent, safe visitations with these individuals. Alternatively, if the FBA revealed the foster child ran away to escape the restrictive nature of the group home, the BCBA and social worker made efforts to involve the youth in determining a preferred type of living situation or setting. Compared with the matched-control group, those who had received FBA-informed interventions ran away from their foster care placement significantly fewer times. In sum, this prevention strategy decreased placement disruptions for foster children.

Case Study 2

During the course of the authors' clinical work at APMRT, some problem behaviors have been assessed and treated that may be unique to foster youth. As a particular challenging example, the authors served Donatello, an 8-year-old boy diagnosed with ADHD, who was placed in a foster home with 3 additional foster children. His case manager referred him for behavioral services due to aggression, noncompliance, and peculiar nighttime behavior. Although Donatello was taking psychotropic medications to address symptoms of ADHD, his foster mother reported his problem behavior was severe at night. Specifically, Donatello roamed the foster house, took items from the fridge, and then hid the items in various locations in his room. This behavior was disruptive to other residents of the home. In particular, Donatello's behavior was stressful to the foster parent, whose sleep often was disrupted by Donatello's nocturnal activities. Notably, Donatello's problem behavior likely was engendered by the neglect he had experienced, which included having limited access to food for extended periods of time. According to data collected by the foster parent during the initial assessment, Donatello never stayed in his room throughout an entire night

(**Fig. 3**). In turn, nighttime foraging gave rise to daytime behavioral issues, such as sleeping in school. The APMRT members developed a multifaceted intervention to both prevent and respond to nighttime food foraging and hoarding.

To reduce Donatello's motivation to seek out food at night, his foster mother gave him protein bars, crackers, and water to keep in his room each night. She also removed most of the toys from his room and placed a motion-detector alarm outside of the door. If Donatello remained in his room throughout the night, the foster parent provided Donatello a sticker and a preferred food item. After Donatello earned a specified number of stickers, he was permitted to select an outing to his favorite restaurant. If Donatello attempted to leave his room during the night, the alarm went off and alerted the foster mother, who then escorted Donatello back to his room. In addition, he did not earn a sticker or food item in the morning. With this treatment package, as indicated in **Fig. 3**, Donatello stayed in his bedroom most nights. The success of this intervention likely contributed to Donatello remaining in the same foster care placement for more than a year. Thereafter, he was reunified with his biological family. Without behavioral services, it is possible that Donatello's nighttime foraging and hoarding would have disrupted Donatello's residential placement and further altered his developmental trajectory.

Skill Acquisition Procedures

Because many foster youth have a history of traumatic and neglectful experiences, it is not surprising that they enter the child welfare system with deficits in academic skills[29] and independent living skills.[30] Presumably, if foundational skills, such as appropriate social interactions, fluent reading and comprehension, and basic adaptive skills, are not taught, foster youth transitioning into adulthood may not have the necessary prerequisite skills to enable them to be successful, contributing members of a community.[31] BCBAs are well equipped to design teaching procedures to ensure that foster care settings promote healthy life skills.

During the course of the project, the authors found that many foster parents incorrectly assume that foster children have age-appropriate skill sets. For example, foster parents may become upset when a 9-year-old foster child does not shower, brush her teeth, or wear clean clothes and, likewise, urinates in her bed each night. Foster

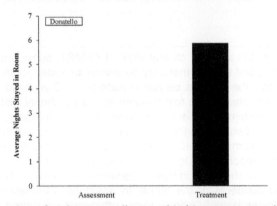

Fig. 3. Average number of nights Donatello stayed in his room per week across a 7-month period. Note that nighttime roaming that often resulted in hoarding food items. During the assessment phase (first week), Donatello consistently did not stay in his room at night. Following the implementation of a function-based treatment (next 22 weeks), Donatello spent most nights in his room without foraging.

parents often report frustration with what they perceive as the youth's willful noncompliance or disrespect and, consequently, some foster parents have requested the removal of the foster child from their home. To prevent these types of placement disruptions, BCBAs work with foster parents to implement evidence-based skill acquisition procedures to teach various skills to foster children. As a part of this practice, the authors teach foster parents to recognize skill deficits in foster children that result from nonsupportive (neglectful) environments. Behavioral skill acquisition procedures, often used with individuals with intellectual disabilities and neurodevelopmental disorders, typically consist of assessing the skill prior to intervention, breaking down the skill into discrete steps, providing frequent opportunities to practice the skill, and responding consistently to correct and incorrect responses.[31,32]

For example, researchers evaluated the extent to which a multicomponent treatment package increased the number of weeks 2 foster youth slept through the night without urinary accidents.[33] The components included a contingency contract, removal of pull-ups, and a clean-up procedure. Based on outcomes of a preference assessment, the caregiver and child created a written agreement (ie, contingency contract) outlining items the child would earn for achieving a daily goal, a weekly goal, and a bonus goal. Practitioners created goals based on data collected by the caregiver prior to the intervention. Briefly, if the child was dry in the morning and thus met the daily goal, the caregiver delivered the daily goal reward when the child awoke. If the child's behavior met the weekly goal or bonus goal, the caregiver provided the contracted item at that time. If the child had a urinary accident, the caregiver reviewed the accident with the child on waking up and prompted the child to remove the linen and place it in the washing machine. The multicomponent package was successful in decreasing bed-wetting within 7 weeks. At a 3-month follow-up, caregivers did not record any bed-wetting. Notably, there are pharmacologic interventions (eg, imipramine and desmopressin acetate) to treat the symptoms of bed-wetting.[34] After prescribers discontinue the medications, however, enuresis often returns. Thus, pharmacologic interventions for bed-wetting may not be a long-term solution.[35] Altogether, behavioral skill acquisition procedures not only promote the development of skills but also promote the longevity of results.

Case Study 3

Based on the authors' experience, challenging behaviors displayed by foster youth often are indicative of skill deficits. Jax was a 16-year old boy with a variety of diagnoses (oppositional defiant disorder, ADHD, bipolar disorder, and mild intellectual disability). According to his foster parent, he often would drag on when she asked him to complete chores or self-care tasks, such as washing his face and brushing his teeth. In addition to frustrating his foster parents, Jax's deficient self-care skills also affected his interactions with peers. As shown in **Fig. 4**, when the BCBA asked Jax to wash his face, he did so with low independence (ie, he needed considerable guidance). Given these data, the BCBA developed a skill acquisition procedure in which each step of face washing was segmented in discrete units with a picture and textual description. During the teaching phase, the BCBA read and modeled the steps. The BCBA then asked Jax to practice the skill. When he did so independently, the BCBA praised him and offered Jax a preferred snack. During follow-up, the therapist asked Jax to complete the task without any supports. Jax continued to wash his face with high levels of independence. The BCBA taught Jax multiple self-care skills with similar procedures. In short, Jax had multiple skill deficits that were likely a byproduct of the neglect he experienced. The authors addressed these deficits with specific behavioral teaching procedures.

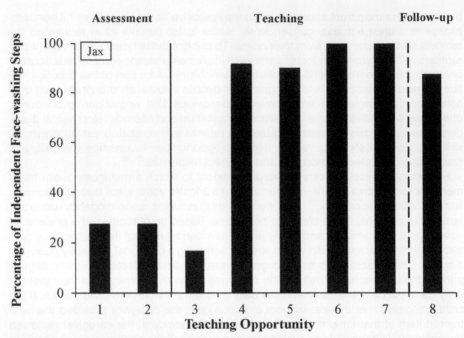

Fig. 4. A graphic depiction of Jax's progress to wash his face over a 4-month period. During the assessment phase (first month), Jax did not complete this task with high levels of independence. When BCBAs and their assistants implemented a skill acquisition procedure of instructions, modeling, and pictorial representations of the steps to complete face washing. This was maintained at a follow-up appointment without the use of additional supports.

Parent Training

Foster parents can be powerful agents in enhancing the lives of foster youth who reside in their homes; foster parents trained in behavioral interventions may have an incomprehensible influence on a child's immediate and future life.[36] Similar to the youth in their care, foster parents also need evidence-based instruction about how to (1) best respond to challenging behaviors displayed by foster children and (2) optimally arrange their homes to encourage and teach critical skills to foster children. If parents respond in a therapeutic and consistent manner when disruptive behavior occurs, a child may display lower levels of disruptive behavior, which, in turn, should result in fewer placement disruptions. As such, the child could spend more time in a school and home environment interacting with teachers and parents who prompt, encourage, and affirm appropriate behavior.

One training strategy, behavioral skills training (BST), is an empirically supported method to teach caregivers to implement behavioral interventions.[37] BST typically includes instruction, modeling, rehearsal, and feedback. First, the BCBA provides instructions (either presented in a written and/or vocal format) that describe the intervention, provides a rationale for the intervention, and outlines the steps of the intervention. Second, the BCBA models the target skill by conducting a simulated session in which the parent pretends to be a foster child and the BCBA demonstrates the intervention. Third, the BCBA requires the parent to practice or rehearse the intervention under her supervision. If possible, the BCBA may simulate a foster child's behavior while the parent implements the intervention. Finally, the BCBA delivers positive performance feedback to the parent by indicating the steps of the intervention conducted correctly and providing corrective feedback for steps performed incorrectly. The BCBA continues the rehearsal and feedback components until the parent correctly implements the intervention in a training context at a mastery level (typically 90% correct implementation of the intervention components across 3 practice opportunities). Upon mastery, the parent implements the behavioral strategy with the foster child while the BCBA supervises and provides feedback as needed.

As a whole, studies show that BST increases (1) foster parents' ability to assess and identify appropriate behavioral interventions,[38] (2) residential staff members' level of positive interactions with residents,[39,40] and (3) group home staff members' accuracy when using a problem solving strategies with foster youth.[41] Furthermore, at least 1 study shows that biological parents whom BCBAs had trained to implement behavioral strategies were reunified more frequently with their children than those who did not participate in the experiential parent training courses.[42]

More broadly, 2 foster parent curricula (ie, Parenting Tools for Positive Behavior Change and Tools of Choice, based on Glenn Latham's book, *The Power of Positive Parenting*[43]) have been developed to teach behavioral interventions to foster parents and biological parents.[42,44,45] Researchers evaluated the extent to which a 30-hour training, which was based on the latter curriculum, and weekly in-home visits with a BCBA increased 163 foster parents' accuracy when implementing interventions during role-play assessments.[44] The researchers designed these role-play assessments to simulate scenarios foster parents frequently encountered with youth (eg, 2 foster youth playing and arguing while playing video games).

After preintervention assessments, researchers used group-delivered instruction at each class to review a target skill (eg, giving positive consequences to the child). In addition, a BCBA visited the foster home for 1-hour weekly appointments for several weeks. During these visits, the BCBA worked with parents to refine the skills taught in the class that week. Following completion of the 30-hour course and weekly in-home appointments, participants' scores improved for each of the targeted skills. Furthermore, parents also implemented the behavioral interventions with their foster child in the home with high levels of accuracy, suggesting that skills taught in classes translated directly to working with their children.[44]

Case Study 4

As a multidisciplinary team, the authors aim to cultivate therapeutic environments for foster youth. One such way is to ensure foster parents receive evidence-based training to best prevent and respond to problem behavior. As an example, the authors treated Gavin, a 7-year-old boy, who was referred for hitting, property destruction, and screaming. As indicated by the pre–parent training phase in **Fig. 5**, Gavin's destructive behavior occurred at high levels, and the foster parent did not consistently implement therapeutic practices like contingent praise, concise directives, and appropriate redirection. Following a training package that included BST, Gavin's foster mother implemented these strategies at a higher level (indicated in the post–parent training phase). The red circle in **Fig. 5** (in the post–parent training phase) denotes when the foster parents implemented the intervention plan with lower levels of accuracy for the first time. Accordingly, Gavin's problem behavior rapidly escalated. This outcome illustrates the importance of adhering to interventions plans, particularly during the early part of the behavior-change process. These data reveal the importance of foster parents consistently and correctly applying behavioral interventions to reduce challenging behavior. Although the long-term impact of this intervention has yet to be determined, it is clear

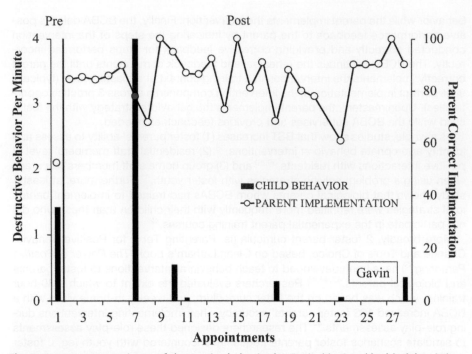

Fig. 5. Responses per minute of destructive behavior by Gavin (depicted by black bars) during 90-minute appointments across a 6-month period. Gavin's foster mother's correct implementation of evidence-based behavioral is depicted with the white circles pre–parent training (Pre) and post–parent training (Post). As indicated by the red circle, the first lapse or errors in the intervention from the foster mother were associated with an increase in Gavin's destructive behavior.

the immediate outcome has allowed for more opportunities for Gavin to interact positively with his foster mother, likely strengthening alternative, appropriate behaviors.

RECOMMENDATIONS FOR PEDIATRICIANS

When visiting with foster youth and their families during appointments, the authors strongly recommend that pediatricians encourage foster care providers and parents to use practices based on the science of behavior. This is important particularly when caring for children with disruptive behavior (eg, aggression, tantrums, hoarding, and bed-wetting). The APMRT develops systems to monitor psychotropic medication use while also using behavioral assessments and interventions for foster youth in Alabama (see Luna and colleagues[46] for a project description). As a part of the authors' prevention strategies, their team has created and uploaded free electronic resources (eg, brief videos and documents; see https://cla.auburn.edu/apmrt/foster-parents/) detailing empirically supported interventions for foster youth. Modules include instruction on day and nighttime toilet training, teaching self-care skills and chores, and consistent use of routines. In addition, the authors provide resources surrounding the influence of traumatic events on problem behavior. To prevent problems that stem from long-term use of psychotropic medication, the authors also encourage pediatricians treating foster youth to be familiar with state-funded groups who monitor the use of psychotropic medications and provide medication review services (eg, APMRT, Ohio Minds Matter, and Texas STAR Health). With state and federal emphasis on multidisciplinary teams, the authors are optimistic about the future of children within the child welfare system.

DISCLOSURE

John T. Rapp (second author) receives funding for the Alabama Psychiatric Medication Review Team from the Alabama Department of Human Resources, Family Services Division.

REFERENCES

1. United States Department of Health and Human Services, Administration for Children and Families, Administration on Children, Youth and Families, Children's Bureau. The AFCARS report: preliminary FY 2016 estimates as of Oct 20, 2017 (No. 24). Washington, DC: Research and Evaluation, Administration for Children and Families, US Department of Health and Human Services; 2017. Available at: https://www.acf.hhs.gov/sites/default/files/cb/afcarsreport24.pdf.
2. US Department of Health and Human Services. Federal definition of foster care and related terms. 2000. Available at: https://www.dhs.state.mn.us/main/groups/county_access/documents/pub/dhs_id_027331.pdf.
3. Bronsard G, Alessandrini M, Fond G, et al. The prevalence of mental disorders among children and adolescents in the child welfare system: A systematic review and meta-analysis. Medicine 2016;95:1–17.
4. Williams CA. Mentoring and social skills training: Ensuring better outcomes for youth in foster care. Child Welfare 2011;90:59–74.
5. United States Government Accountability Office. Children's mental health: concerns remain about appropriate services for children in medicaid and foster care. GAO-13-15. Washington, DC: United States Government Accountability Office; 2012. Available at: http://www.gao.gov/assets/660/650716.pdf.
6. Leathers SJ. Foster children's behavioral disturbance and detachment from caregivers and community institutions. Child Youth Serv Rev 2002;24:239–68.
7. Newton RR, Litrownick AJ, Landsverk JA. Children and youth in foster care: Disentangling the relationship between problem behaviors and number of placements. Child Abuse Negl 2000;24:1363–74.
8. Pecora PJ. Maximizing educational achievement of youth in foster care and alumni: Factors associated with success. Child Youth Serv Rev 2012;34:1121–9.
9. Baglivio MT, Epps N, Swartz K, et al. The prevalence of adverse childhood experiences (ACE) in the lives of juvenile offenders. J Juv Justice 2014;3. Available at: http://www.journalofjuvjustice.org/JOJJ0302/article01.htm.
10. King B, Putnam-Hornstein E, Cederbaum JA, et al. A cross-sectional examination of birth rates among adolescent girls in foster care. Child Youth Serv Rev 2014; 36:179–86.
11. Dworsky A, Napolitano L, Courtney M. Homelessness during the transition from foster care to adulthood. Am J Public Health 2013;103:S318–23.
12. Baer DM, Wolf MM, Risley TR. Some current dimensions of applied behavior analysis. J Appl Behav Anal 1968;1:91–7.
13. Skinner BF. Selection by consequences. Science 1981;213:501–4.
14. Child and Family Services Improvement and Innovation Act, 20 U.S.C. § 112-134 (2011) Available at: https://www.congress.gov/112/plaws/publ34/PLAW-112publ34.pdf.

15. Whitehouse CM, Vollmer TR, Colbert B. Evaluating the use of computerized stimulus preference assessments in foster care. J Appl Behav Anal 2014;47:470–84.
16. Parker J. When things go wrong! Placement disruption and termination: Power and student perspectives. Br J Soc Work 2008;40(3):983–99.
17. Zima BT, Bussing R, Crecelius GM, et al. Psychotropic medication treatment patterns among school-aged children in foster care. J Child Adolesc Psychopharmacol 1999;9:135–47.
18. Rubin D, Matone M, Huang YS, et al. Interstate variation in trends of psychotropic medication use among Medicaid-enrolled children in foster care. Child Youth Serv Rev 2012;34:1492–9.
19. Crystal S, Olfson M, Huang C, et al. Broadened use of atypical antipsychotics: safety, effectiveness, and policy challenges. Health Aff 2009;28:w770–81.
20. U.S. Government Accountability Office. Foster children: HHS guidance could help states improve oversight of psychotropic medications (Publication No. GAO-12-270T). Washington, DC: United States Government Accountability Office; 2011.
21. Stambaugh LF, Leslie LK, Ringeisen H, et al. Psychotropic medication use by children in child welfare. OPRE Report #2012-33. Washington, DC: Office of Planning, Research and Evaluation, Administration for Children and Families, U.S. Department of Health and Human Services; 2012.
22. Singh AN, Matson JL, Mouttapa M, et al. A critical item analysis of the QABF: development of a short form assessment instrument. Res Dev Disabil 2009;30: 782–92.
23. Hanley GP. Functional assessment of problem behavior: Dispelling myths, overcoming implementation obstacles, and developing new lore. Behav Anal Pract 2012;5:54–72.
24. Vollmer TR, Borrero JC, Wright CS, et al. Identifying possible contingencies during descriptive analyses of severe behavior disorders. J Appl Behav Anal 2001; 34:269–87.
25. Iwata BA, Dozier CL. Clinical application of functional analysis methodology. Behav Anal Pract 2008;1:3–9.
26. Gresham FM, Watson TS, Skinner CH. Functional behavioral assessment: principles, procedures, and future directions. Sch Psychol Rev 2001;30:156–72.
27. Clark HB, Crosland KA, Geller D, et al. A functional approach to reducing runaway behavior and stabilizing placements for adolescents in foster care. Res Soc Work Pract 2008;18:429–41.
28. Ingram K, Lewis-Palmer T, Sugai G. Function-based intervention planning: comparing the effectiveness of FBA function-based and non-function based intervention plans. J Posit Behav Interv 2005;7:224–36.
29. Pears KC, Heywood CV, Kim HK, et al. Prereading deficits in children in foster care. Sch Psychol Rev 2011;40:140–8.
30. Leathers SJ, Testa MF. Foster youth emancipating from care: caseworkers' reports on needs and services. Child Welfare 2006;85:463–98.
31. Courtney ME, Piliavin I, Grogan-Kaylor A, et al. Foster youth transitions to adulthood: a longitudinal view of youth leaving care. Child Welfare 2001;80:685.
32. Kurtz PF, Lind MA. Behavioral approaches to treatment of intellectual and developmental disabilities. In: Madden G, editor. APA Handbook of Behavior Analysis, volume 2, Applied/Clinical Issues. Washington, DC: American Psychological Association; 2013. p. 279–99.
33. Stover AC, Dunlap G, Neff B. The effects of a contingency contracting program on the nocturnal enuresis of three children. Res Soc Work Pract 2008;18:421–8.

34. Thurber S. Childhood enuresis: current diagnostic formulations, salient findings, and effective treatment modalities. Arch Psychiatr Nurs 2017;31:319–23.
35. Cendron M. Primary nocturnal enuresis: current concepts. Am Fam Physician 1999;59:1205–24.
36. Greeno EJ, Lee BR, Uretsky MC, et al. Effects of a foster parent training intervention on child behavior, caregiver stress, and parenting style. J Child Fam Stud 2016;25:1991–2000.
37. Conklin SM, Wallace MD. Pyramidal parent training using behavioral skills training: Training caregivers in the use of a differential reinforcement procedure. Behav Interv 2019;37:377–87.
38. Shayne R, Miltenberger RG. Evaluation of behavioral skills training for teaching functional assessment and treatment selection skills to parents. Behav Interv 2013;28:4–21.
39. Crosland KA, Dunlap G, Sager W, et al. The effects of staff training on the types of interactions observed at two group homes for foster care children. Res Soc Work Pract 2008;18:410–20.
40. McDougale CB, Coon JC, Richling SM, et al. Group procedures for decreasing problem behavior displayed by detained adolescents. Behav Modif 2019;43(5): 615–38.
41. Skelton E, Crosland KA, Clark HBR. Acquisition of a social problem-solving method by caregivers in the foster care system: Evaluation and implications. Child Fam Behav Ther 2016;38:32–46.
42. Franks SB, Mata FC, Wofford E, et al. The effects of behavioral parent training on placement outcomes of biological families in a state child welfare system. Res Soc Work Pract 2013;23:377–82.
43. Latham GI. The power of positive parenting. North Logan (UT): P&T Ink; 1994.
44. Van Camp CM, Vollmer TR, Goh HL, et al. Behavioral parent training in child welfare: evaluations of skills acquisition. Res Soc Work Pract 2008;18:377–91.
45. Van Camp CM, Montgomery JL, Vollmer TR, et al. Behavioral parent training in child welfare: maintenance and booster training. Res Soc Work Pract 2008;18: 392–400.
46. Luna O, Rapp JT, Newland MC, et al. Alabama psychiatric medication review team (APMRT): Advocating for foster children. Behav Soc Issues 2018;AA16–20. https://doi.org/10.5210/bsi.v.27i0.8298.

Pediatric Prevention
Feeding Disorders

Vivian F. Ibañez, PhD, BCBA-D[a],*, Kathryn M. Peterson, PhD, BCBA-D[a],
Jaime G. Crowley, PhD, BCBA-D[b], Sarah D. Haney, PhD, BCBA[c],
Ashley S. Andersen, MS, BCBA[c], Cathleen C. Piazza, PhD, BCBA-D[d]

KEYWORDS

- Applied behavior analysis • Avoidant and restrictive food intake disorder
- Food refusal • Food selectivity • Pediatric feeding disorder • Pediatric prevention

KEY POINTS

- The systematic, data-based approach that behavior analysts use is well established and ideal to identify the variables that influence mealtime behavior and to prescribe an intervention based on those identified variables.
- Preintervention interdisciplinary evaluation is indicated to establish the safety of oral feeding and rule out medical causes of the feeding disorder, given that the cause of most feeding disorders is multifactorial.
- Although many children will "grow out" of their feeding problems, early intervention is critical for those children whose feeding problems persist to establish and maintain the developmental progression of feeding skills. In some cases, pediatricians may need to refer children with severe feeding disorders to an intensive feeding program that provides goal-oriented, data-based assessment and intervention.
- Common general strategies that behavior analysts use with children with feeding disorders are to reduce the effort of feeding, to maximize caregiver attention for appropriate feeding behavior, and to minimize attention and coaxing for inappropriate mealtime behavior.
- Diagnosis, referral, and management of pediatric feeding disorders represent excellent areas for partnerships between pediatricians and behavior analysts who specialize in intervention of pediatric feeding disorders. Early recognition of a feeding disorder is critical to provide recommendations to caregivers or to make referrals for appropriate services.

[a] Children's Specialized Hospital and Rutgers University, 200 Somerset St, New Brunswick, NJ 08901, USA; [b] May Institute, 41 Pacella Park Dr, Randolph, MA 02368, USA; [c] University of Nebraska Medical Center's Munroe-Meyer Institute, 42nd and Emile, Omaha, NE 68198, USA; [d] Rutgers University Graduate School of Applied and Professional Psychology and Children's Specialized Hospital, 152 Frelinghuysen Road, Piscataway, NJ 08854, USA
* Corresponding author.
E-mail address: vivian.ibanez@rutgers.edu

Pediatr Clin N Am 67 (2020) 451–467
https://doi.org/10.1016/j.pcl.2020.02.003
0031-3955/20/© 2020 Elsevier Inc. All rights reserved.

INTRODUCTION

Most adults give little thought to the mechanics of eating, a routine activity that occurs many times a day in many places with many different people across the lifespan. Nevertheless, successful eating requires coordination of a chain of behaviors, and this behavior chain has significant effects on a child's growth, development, and socialization. Physical growth, in fact, is a common proxy for feeding behavior that pediatricians use to evaluate an infant's health and well-being. Feeding also sets the occasion for infant and caregiver bonding and for meaningful social interactions between the child and caregivers, other adults, and peers. Persistent feeding problems, such as insufficient intake of calories or nutrition, therefore, can have short- and long-term negative consequences on a child's behavior, health, and socialization.[1,2] Children whose diets are high in fat, salt, sugar, or a combination are at risk for severe health problems such as obesity, type-2 diabetes, chronic constipation, and hypertension.[1,3] Children who rely solely on oral consumption of fluids or receive most calories via enteral or parenteral nutrition may not have sufficient opportunities to practice feeding skills. Caregivers of children with feeding disorders report feelings of rejection, anxiety, depression, an inability to bond with their children, low confidence, and stress.[4–7] Young children may be at greatest risk for the negative health consequences of a feeding disorder, as the most damaging effects of inadequate calories, poor nutrition, or both occur before age 5 years, which is a period of critical brain development.[8] Therefore, early identification and management of feeding disorders is important for preventing or mitigating its short- and long-term negative consequences. The aims of the current paper are (1) to describe how to recognize feeding disorders, (2) to discuss the environmental variables that may cause and maintain feeding disorders, and (3) to provide recommendations for prevention and intervention for feeding disorders based on the applied behavior-analytic research literature.

DEFINITION

Many caregivers will raise concerns about their child's feeding behavior during well-child visits. These problems tend to be transient, however, and will resolve without intervention.[9,10] Nevertheless, some children have persistent feeding problems that do not resolve without intervention.[11] For example, Esparo and colleagues[12] questioned the caregivers of 851 children and found that 4.8% of children had persistent feeding problems, defined as chronic difficulties with eating at a developmentally appropriate level and growth concerns (eg, weight loss) for at least 1 month. The challenge for pediatricians, therefore, is to determine which problems are transient and which require intervention (**Box 1**).

Weight Gain and Growth

Although plotting serial weight gain and growth provides an objective measure of growth relative to a child's same-age and same-sex peers, determining whether an

---

Box 1
Indications of a feeding disorder and need for intervention

Child has 3 consecutive months of weight loss

Child is diagnosed with dehydration, which results in emergency intervention

Child has nasogastric, gastrostomy, or jejunostomy tube with no increase in oral calories, fluids, or both for 3 consecutive months

individual child's growth is faltering may be challenging. The pediatrician must consider the child's gestational age; genetic, metabolic, or other physical problems that affect growth; serial growth rate; and parental height to better predict the child's growth potential. Confirmation that the caregiver is presenting adequate calories and obtaining an estimate of the child's caloric intake also is critical. Weight loss despite the availability of adequate calories is a cause for intervention.[13–15] Other indications for intervention include insufficient fluid intake that requires emergency-room or critical-care visits for rehydration.[16]

Enteral Feeding

Nasogastric, gastrostomy, and jejunostomy tubes are tools to promote weight gain and growth until a child is able or willing to consume calories and fluids orally,[9] given that the child is safe for oral feeding. Although most children transition from enteral to oral feeding, many do not without therapy.[17] Hoogewerfand colleagues[18] found that children who required enteral feedings for more than 30 days were likely to need intervention to transition successfully to oral feeding.

Developmental Progression of Feeding

Feeding disorders are difficult to identify because their characteristics are heterogeneous and may include refusal to eat foods or drink liquids, refusal to eat specific types or textures of food, dependence on a limited or developmentally inappropriate source of nutrition, and refusal to self-feed or transition to age- or developmentally appropriate textures.[19] **Table 1** shows a comparison of the typical developmental sequence of feeding behavior relative to a disorder pattern of feeding behavior, which is one method for recognizing disordered feeding. Note that even typical feeding behavior is not perfectly consistent and may vary in quality or quantity.

Caregiver Concerns

Some caregiver concerns about child feeding behavior are a function of misperception.[20] In these cases, support and education will alleviate caregiver concerns, as many children will "grow out" of their feeding problems. However, pediatricians should consider whether a child has an emerging feeding disorder when typical strategies do not alleviate caregiver concerns. In some cases, pediatricians might assume that the distress a caregiver demonstrates or the unusual feeding practices he or she uses is the cause of the child's feeding problem; however, it might be that the child's feeding problem is the cause of the caregiver's distress and his or her adoption of unusual feeding practices. For example, in the authors' clinical practice, they observe that most caregivers of children with feeding disorders spend an unusually long time trying to get their child to feed, just to ensure that the child is consuming adequate calories for growth. As a general guideline, meal lengths greater than 30 minutes are one of the best indicators of a feeding disorder.

CAUSE AND EVALUATION

Feeding disorders may develop and persist because of anatomic, neurodevelopmental, oral-motor, medical, and environmental factors that occur in isolation or in combination.[11,15] Feeding behavior (eg, sucking, chewing) improves with practice. Thus, inadequate oral-feeding experience (eg, due to prematurity or enteral feeds) limits opportunities to practice the feeding skills that are necessary for the child to become an efficient and effective oral feeder.[19,21] Limited oral-feeding experience also limits pairings of internal experiences of hunger and the satiety that occurs after an oral feed.[13]

Table 1
A developmental comparison of typical and disordered feeding

Age (Months)	Feeding Behavior	Typical	Disordered
Birth	Nipple feeding	Accepts	Has difficulty
	Suck-swallow-breathe	Coordinated	Uncoordinated
		Improves over time	Does not improve over time
	Signals when hungry	Cries	Cries inconsistently
	Quality and quantity of feeds	Consistent	Best while sleeping
4–6	Baby food	Accepts	Rejects or inconsistently accepts
	Tongue thrust	Decreases	Persists
	Lateral tongue movements	Emerge	Do not emerge or are inconsistent
12	Mashed table food	Accepts	Does not accept, coughs, gags
18	Picky eating emerges for children with typical and disordered feeding		
	Previously refused foods	Will eat with consistent exposure	Will not eat
	Food variety	Eats many foods	Eats only a few foods
	Meets caloric needs from food	Meets	Does not meet or are excessive
	Meets nutritional needs from food	Meets	Does not meet
	Fluid intake	Adequate	Inadequate
36	Chewing skills	Rotary chew emerges	Immature pattern, munching, uses tongue to push food against hard palate
		Consistently chews and masticates a variety of food textures	Eats meltable solids (eg, cookies, chips) and purees (eg, applesauce, mashed potatoes, yogurt) primarily
	Meal length	20–30 min	More than 30 min
	Choking, coughing, gagging	Minimal	Occurs periodically or often
	Food pocketing	Minimal	Occurs periodically or often
School Age	Social influences on feeding	Influenced by peers	Not influenced by peers
	Change disrupts feeding	No	Yes
	Response to hunger	Will eat nonpreferred food	Will not eat nonpreferred food

Children with limited oral-feeding experience may have difficulty swallowing; propelling the bolus toward the pharynx; lateralizing the tongue; closing the lips around the teat, cup, or utensil; retaining the bolus in the mouth; and chewing, to name a few.[22–24] These children may not manage age- or developmentally appropriate textures.

Medical Conditions

Children with medical conditions such as gastroesophageal reflux disease might associate feeding with the pain caused by eruption of acidic stomach contents into the esophagus[25,26] and cry and refuse feedings to avoid pain. However, feeding disorders may persist long after medical intervention alleviates the condition.[27–29] For

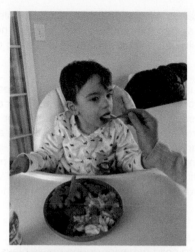

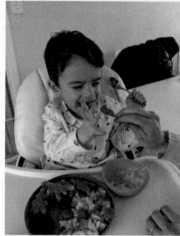

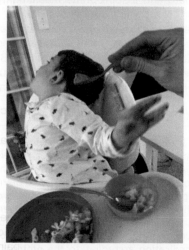

example, Nelson and colleagues[30] showed that feeding problems persisted even after gastroesophageal-reflux symptoms resolved. **Fig. 1** shows how an unidentified food allergy or intolerance could cause or contribute to a feeding disorder.

Oral-Motor-Skill Deficits

Similarly, a child who refuses to feed because feeding causes pain does not practice the skills necessary to become an effective oral feeder. Other children have underlying oral-motor-skill deficits, such as dysphagia, or anatomic or craniofacial conditions, such as hypotonia or Pierre-Robin sequence, that negatively affect oral-feeding skills. Failure to develop appropriate oral-motor skills or oral-motor-skill dysfunction contributes to unpleasant feeding experiences. That is, poor oral-motor skills increase the likelihood the child will choke or gag or that feeding is "hard work" because the child does not or cannot coordinate feeding behavior such as the suck-swallow-breathe response.

Caregiver Behavior

How caregivers respond to child behavior during meals plays an important role in the persistence of a feeding disorder.[31–33] In their clinical practice, the authors commonly observe that caregivers will try many things to encourage their child to eat, such as providing escape from the meal (eg, removing the bite, ending the meal), coaxing (eg, "These carrots are good for you!"), or providing the child with a preferred food or toy.[34] Although most caregivers use such responses with their typically eating children with no or limited negative effects, these consequences often worsen the mealtime behavior of children with feeding disorders.[32,33] Borrero and colleagues[34] showed that the most common caregiver responses to child's inappropriate mealtime behavior were removing the bite or drink or ending the meal and providing attention, such as coaxing (eg, "You like peas"). Piazza and colleagues[32] also observed caregivers give their child a preferred food to ensure the child consumed something during the meal or a toy or activity to calm or distract the child.

Functional Analysis

Applied behavior analysts have evaluated how these caregiver responses during meals affect the appropriate and inappropriate mealtime behavior of children with feeding disorders using a test called *functional analysis*.[32,33] A functional analysis of inappropriate mealtime behavior measures how specific caregiver responses to inappropriate mealtime behavior affect child behavior. The caregiver responses that the functional analysis tests are based on studies like that of Borrero and colleagues[34] and Piazza and colleagues[32] that have observed and documented how caregivers are likely to respond to child's inappropriate mealtime behavior. The responses the

Fig. 1. This figure shows how pain or discomfort paired with feeding can cause or contribute to the development of a feeding disorder. Caregivers reported that Fred used to eat most foods without any problems when they fed him. They noticed, however, that certain foods they subsequently added to Fred's diet caused diarrhea, skin rash, and vomiting. Fred began crying and pushing the spoon away when his caregivers fed him. Fred's oral intake decreased despite the caregivers' efforts. Fred's caregivers called their pediatrician who referred them to a gastroenterologist. The gastroenterologist diagnosed Fred with eosinophilic esophagitis. Even though Fred's caregivers removed suspected allergens from Fred's diet and used his medication according to the prescription, his feeding behavior did not improve. Fred even refused to eat foods that he used to eat without any problems.

functional analysis tests are brief escape from bite or drink presentations (ie, the feeder removes the bite or drink) in the *escape* condition; adult attention (eg, the adult coaxes the child) in the *attention* condition; or access to a tangible item, such as a preferred food, toy, or activity, in the *tangible* condition. The *control* condition, during which the feeder interacts with the child and does not respond to child's inappropriate mealtime behavior, serves as a comparison for the escape, attention, and tangible conditions.[32] Research on pediatric feeding disorders has shown that rates of inappropriate mealtime behavior tend to be highest when inappropriate mealtime behavior produces escape from bite or drink presentations, and many children with feeding disorders will have inappropriate mealtime behavior when it produces adult attention. Said another way, although caregivers remove bites or drinks or provide attention following inappropriate mealtime behavior with the goal of encouraging the child to eat, these consequences do not increase the likelihood the child will eat and increase the likelihood the child will engage in inappropriate mealtime behavior. Thus, results of studies on the functional analysis of inappropriate mealtime behavior show that children with feeding disorders often have inappropriate mealtime behavior to get out of eating and to get adult attention.

INTERDISCIPLINARY EVALUATION

Taken together, a child's failure or inability to eat and drink by mouth is typically caused by a complex interaction between many factors. For this reason, interdisciplinary assessment is important to rule out, treat, or address medical, oral-motor, and nutritional issues before beginning feeding therapy (**Table 2**). Ongoing consultation from the interdisciplinary team may be necessary to treat emergent medical problems (eg, food allergy), maintain the child's safety for oral feeding, and ensure that the child's diet is calorically and nutritionally appropriate.[29,35–37]

DATA COLLECTION

Caregiver report is likely the most common way that pediatricians obtain information about problematic feeding behavior. Research shows, however, that vocal report based on recollection may not be an accurate representation of child behavior.[38] Therefore, the authors present an alternative and potentially less biased method of obtaining information in the next section.

Table 2
Potential interdisciplinary team members who might evaluate a child with a feeding

Interdisciplinary Feeding Team Member	Role
Behavior Analyst with feeding expertise	Assess the contribution of environmental variables to the child's feeding disorder
Dietitian	Evaluate the child's caloric and nutritional needs and monitor growth and hydration
Physician	Rule out medical causes of the feeding disorder
Psychology or Social Worker	Evaluate family stressors, recruit resources for the family
Swallowing Expert • Occupational Therapist • Speech and Language Pathologist	Evaluate oral-motor skills, swallow safety, and the need for adaptive equipment: identify appropriate food textures and bolus sizes

Table 3
A simple data sheet for collecting meal start and stop times

	Breakfast		AM Snack		Lunch		PM Snack		Dinner	
Date	Start	Stop	Start	Stop	Start	Stop	Start	Stop	Start	Stop
3/12/2020	7:00	7:45	10:00	11:00	1:00	2:15	3:00	3:45	5:00	6:30
3/13/2020	9:00	10:20	12:00	1:15	3:00	3:45	4:30	5:10	7:00	8:30
3/14/2020	6:00	7:30	9:20	10:15	1:00	2:30	3:15	4:00	6:00	7:15
3/15/2020	8:15	9:30	12:20	1:00	2:30	3:15	4:15	5:15	6:15	7:30
3/16/2020	7:15	8:45	10:30	11:45	1:00	2:45	3:30	4:15	5:00	6:45

The sample data show that the child's meal lengths are long, and the child has an inconsistent meal schedule.

Direct-Observation Data Collection

Direct observation of behavior is a cornerstone of behavioral assessment. Pediatricians do not have the time to observe meals directly, but they can instruct caregivers to collect direct-observation data to better understand a child's feeding disorder. Meal length is a good predictor of a feeding disorder, so having caregivers record meal length can help pediatricians identify problematic feeding behavior. **Table 3** is an example of a simple data sheet on which the caregiver could record the date and the start and stop times for each meal. Start and stop times will provide information about meal length and whether caregivers follow a consistent meal schedule.

Three-Day Food Record			
Date	Food Item (type of food and brand)	Yield	Amount Consumed
1/14/19	Eggo waffles	2 waffles	½ waffle
	Publix chocolate milk	¼ cup	¼ cup
	Simple Truth chicken sausage link	2 links	¼ link
	Mashed banana	1 banana	¼ banana
1/14/19	5 Tyson chicken nuggets	5 nuggets	3 nuggets
	Publix chocolate milk	1 cup	½ cup
	Lay's plain potato chips	1 bag	1 bag
	Cotton candy grapes	12 grapes	2 grapes
1/14/19	Famous Amos chocolate chip cookies	8 cookies	4 cookies
	Water	1 cup	¼ cup
	Gerber Stage 2 chicken and rice	1 cup	1/3 cup
1/14/19	Tyson's Grilled & Ready chicken breast strips	6 pieces	1 piece
	Publix canned green beans	½ cup	None
	Publix canned yellow corn	1 cup	¼ cup
	Annie's white cheddar macaroni & cheese	2 cups	2 cups
	Publix chocolate milk	1 cup	½ cup
	Water	1 cup	None
	Dannon Danimals strawberry smoothie		

Fig. 2. An example of a caregiver-reported food record for 1 day.

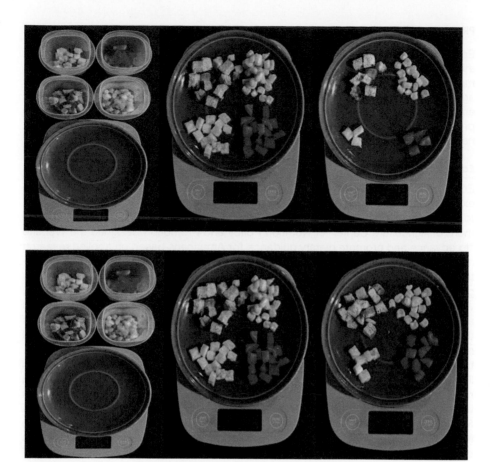

Fig. 3. An example of pre- and postmeal photographs with different amounts consumed.

Food diaries are another method researchers have used to collect data on caloric and nutritional intake. An ideal food record would include the foods served and the pre- and postmeal food weights. A dietitian can calculate caloric and nutritional intake more precisely if the caregiver includes the recipe he or she used to prepare each dish (**Fig. 2**). The recipe also may be helpful if the pediatrician suspects food allergies or intolerances. Caregivers may be unlikely, however, to use such an effortful data-collection procedure. An alternative method is for caregivers to photograph the presented food pre- and postmeal (**Fig. 3**). This method provides less detail but gives a general idea of the child's intake with less effort for the caregiver.

Baseline Data

Evaluating a child's response to intervention systematically after establishing a baseline level of behavior is another characteristic of behavioral assessment. For example, the caregiver might keep a record of intake for a week before making any changes to the mealtime routine. These data would serve as a baseline from which the caregiver could compare the child's behavior pre- and postintervention to determine if the intervention is effective.

PREVENTION

Early intervention is critical for those children whose feeding problems persist. The authors' clinical experience is that children whose feeding problems disrupt the developmental progression of feeding skills often require intensive therapy to become age-typical feeders. In these cases, feeding skills such as chewing do not always emerge without intervention.[13] Thus, early intervention to maintain the developmental progression of feeding skills will mitigate the intensity and duration of intervention needed for the child to become an age-typical feeder.

Education

Education can often address caregiver concerns about child's feeding behavior.[13] An example of an educational tool that is freely available to the public and relatively easy to use is the Website https://www.choosemyplate.gov/. The United States Department of Agriculture Center for Nutrition Policy and Promotion designed the Website "to advance and promote dietary guidance for Americans based on applied research and analyses on nutrition and consumer economics."[39] A caregiver can obtain an estimate of his or her child's caloric needs using the link https://www.choosemyplate.gov/resources/MyPlatePlan. The link will produce a caloric estimate for the child, which will appear on the screen, after the caregiver inputs the child's age, sex, and activity level. The Website will show recommended portion sizes by food group if the caregiver clicks on the calorie estimate. The site has a plethora of other helpful nutritional information and tips (eg, "healthy eating on a budget"). Guidance on mealtime structure, such as serving meals and snacks at the same time every day and limiting unscheduled, between-meal snacking, and the importance of establishing regularly scheduled sleep and wake times also can be beneficial. However, children with feeding disorders do not always respond to strategies that resolve the transient feeding problems that most children have. In fact, these strategies may worsen the feeding behavior of children with feeding disorders. In these cases, pediatricians can adopt tools that applied behavior analysts commonly use to guide caregivers.

Behavioral Strategies

Common strategies behavior analysts use with children with feeding disorders include reducing the effort of feeding (eg, decreasing bite size),[40] directing caregiver attention to appropriate feeding behavior (eg, the caregiver provides praise when the child eats a bite of food),[41] and minimizing caregiver attention and coaxing for inappropriate mealtime behavior (eg, the caregiver does not make a response when the child complains about eating).[41] No intervention will be effective unless caregivers use it consistently and as directed. Generally, the authors recommend using a systematic approach. That is, caregivers should use one intervention at a time and then add or subtract intervention components to determine whether the intervention component is effective. For example, the caregiver might start by minimizing attention for inappropriate mealtime behavior (eg, make no response when the child says, "I don't like that."). If the child's feeding behavior does not improve after 2 weeks, the caregiver could provide praise each time the child eats a bite of food and continue to make no response to child inappropriate mealtime behavior.

The authors later describe procedures that caregivers could use at home for common feeding problems that emerge along the developmental continuum. Although the procedures described later can be effective, they are not without potential side effects. Persistent feeding problems require consistent intervention using the procedures exactly as described, which is often difficult for most caregivers given their many competing responsibilities. In addition, some children have feeding problems that are so severe or complicated that they simply require intervention by a professional no matter how consistent or how well a caregiver uses an intervention. Thus, consider each child's feeding problems and his or her caregiver's emotional and physical resources before recommending a home program. If in doubt, refer the child for professional intervention.

Breast and Bottle Feeding

An uncoordinated suck-swallow-breathe response and inadequate oral intake are 2 common manifestations of feeding disorders in infancy. Infants with feeding disorders often show little interest in feeding; cry but then do not feed well when the caregiver presents the teat; obtain most calories in the first 5 minutes of the feeding; and feed best while initiating sleep or while sleeping. These infants may benefit from non-nutritive sucking on a pacifier between meals to strengthen the suck-breathe response.[42–49] Caregivers should follow a semi-demand feeding schedule with a relatively short interfeed interval of no more than 3 hours between feeds.[50] Short interfeed intervals reduce the demand on the infant to obtain a large volume in any one feed and allow the caregiver to keep each feed short, not more than 10 minutes initially. Caregivers often want to extend feeds when the infant is feeding well. Although stopping the feed according to a fixed time may seem counterintuitive, allowing the infant to continue feeding for an extended period may increase the risk of fatigue and low intake at the subsequent feed.[51] Infants who have uncoordinated suck-swallow-breathe responses may expend more energy trying to feed than they consume during the feed. Short feeds reduce the energy expenditure of any one meal and mitigate fatigue from longer meals. The caregiver can increase feed length and the interfeeding interval, as the infant better coordinates the suck-swallow-breathe response and becomes a more efficient feeder (ie, volume/time increases).

Pureed Food

Common problems include rejection of pureed food, persistent tongue thrust, and coughing or gagging when the food is not completely smooth. Small, frequent meals reduce the effort and unpleasantness of the feed for the child. The caregiver could start by presenting as few as five bites to the child and ending the meal after he or she has presented the five bites. Similarly, the caregiver could reduce the amount of each bite. For example, instead of heaping the bowl of a baby spoon with food, the caregiver could dip the spoon into the food and present the dipped spoon to the child. The caregiver would increase the number of presented bites or the amount of food on the spoon systematically as the child's feeding behavior improves.

Persistent Tongue Thrust

Persistent tongue thrust will result in the child expelling the food from the mouth, and some children will actively spit food. The caregiver should scoop up the expelled food and put it back in the child's mouth. However, the caregiver should swab the child's mouth with a sponge swab such as a Toothette and present a fresh bite if the child produces excessive saliva with the expelled food.[23] Another strategy for severe tongue thrust is to insert a coated baby spoon with a small bolus of food inside the mouth, rotate the spoon 180° inside the mouth, place the tip of the spoon on the middle of the tongue, and gently slide the spoon toward the lips.[44,52–56] The goal is to deposit the bolus on the middle of the child's tongue such that the child need to only elevate the tongue and propel the bolus toward the pharynx. That is, the procedure

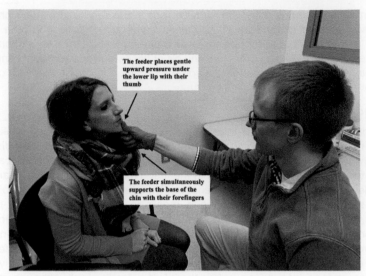

The feeder places gentle upward pressure under the lower lip with their thumb

The feeder simultaneously supports the base of the chin with their forefingers

Fig. 4. Demonstration of the chin-prompt procedure.

eliminates the need for the child to gather food into a bolus and move the bolus to the tongue. Provide caution, however, that too much pressure to the tongue or an incorrectly placed spoon may cause gagging, which could worsen the child's feeding problem.

Open-Mouth Posture

A chin prompt is useful for children with open-mouth posture who do not close their lips around the spoon.[54,57,58] **Fig. 4** shows how the caregiver uses his or her index finger and thumb to prompt the child to close his or her mouth in response to food entering the mouth. The risk of the procedure is that using excessive force during the chin prompt could cause injury and worsen the child's feeding problem. Patience rather than force is the key. For difficult cases, the caregiver should start by presenting only one or a few bites and ending the meal when the child closes his or her mouth. The caregiver then can increase the number of bites presented as the child learns that he or she should close his or her lips around the spoon when the caregiver places the spoon in the child's mouth.

Coughs and Gags

Children who cough and gag when they encounter small lumps in pureed food can benefit from initial presentation of completely smooth food such as Stages 1 and 2 jarred baby food or table food pureed in a smoothie blender.[59] The caregiver then can introduce lumps systematically based on low levels of coughs and gags during feeds.

Tongue Lateralization

Tongue thrust should decrease as tongue lateralization increases. Placing a small amount of sticky food such as peanut butter or honey between the cheek and gums in each quadrant of the child's mouth will encourage the child to lateralize the tongue to retrieve the food. Careful observation is important initially to ensure that the child manages the food safely and does not have an adverse reaction. Caregivers can minimize tooth decay by cleaning the area thoroughly during the child's oral-hygiene routine.

Regular-Textured Food

Munching or an up and down chewing pattern usually emerges as caregivers increase the texture of foods, which is often around 12 months of age. Chewing skills continue to improve, and a relatively mature open-mouth rotary chew should emerge around age 3 years. Children whose chewing skills do not advance should be referred for evaluation. Closed-mouth chewing is often a sign that the child is using his or her tongue to mash food against the hard palate, which is a behavior that likely will interfere with maturation of chewing skills. If the child consumes primarily meltable solids and the child's chewing skills are not maturing, the authors recommend that caregivers stop presenting meltable solids, as these foods tend to encourage the child to use his or her tongue to mash and dissolve the food and interfere with the development of appropriate chewing skills.

Picky Eating

Caregivers often do not realize that exposure is a one important way children develop preferences for foods.[60,61] Thus, caregivers should present foods the child rejects *more* often but in very small amounts. Our culture tends to promote picky eating by only presenting certain foods, such as vegetables, at specific meals (eg, dinner). Thus, limited opportunities to consume these foods decrease the likelihood that individuals develop a preference for the foods via exposure. In the clinic, the authors present foods from every food group at every meal to increase opportunities to consume and to develop a preference for these foods via exposure. Importantly, caregivers should model good eating habits and minimize the availability of foods that are low in nutritional value and high in fat, sodium, and sugar. Caregivers should offer choices but also have rules about eating. The specific rules are often less important than the fact that the caregivers follow through on the rule. For example, a rule might be that each family member must at least taste every food that is served at each meal.

SPECIALIZED BEHAVIORAL FEEDING INTERVENTION

Intensive, data-based feeding programs that use a behavioral approach are appropriate for children who do not respond to traditional therapy or have emergent feeding problems (eg, chronic dehydration requiring hospitalization) that require immediate change. These programs have demonstrated success increasing oral intake, eliminating tube dependency, and preventing tube placement for children at risk.[37,62,63] Kerwin[14] and Volkert and Piazza[15] demonstrated in their reviews of the literature that interventions based on principles of applied behavior analysis were the only ones with empirical support as intervention for pediatric feeding disorders. The systematic, data-based approach that behavior analysts use is ideal to identify the variables that influence mealtime behavior and prescribe an intervention based on those identified variables. In their clinical practice, the authors find that one misconception professionals and caregivers might have is that behavior-analytic–based intervention is only for children with "behavioral" feeding problems. In reality, the cause of feeding disorders that require intensive intervention is multiple and complex. Thus, effective intervention programs must address all the variables that may cause or contribute to the child's feeding disorder. The ultimate goal of these programs is to progress the child to age-typical feeding. Although the path to age-typical eating is individualized for each child, some common goals include increasing caloric intake, increasing acceptance and consumption of solid food and liquids, decreasing supplemental feedings, increasing texture and variety of foods, decreasing inappropriate mealtime behavior, and caregiver training.

SUMMARY

Diagnosis, referral, and management of pediatric feeding disorders represent excellent areas for partnerships between pediatricians and behavior analysts who specialize in intervention of pediatric feeding disorders. Early recognition of a feeding disorder is critical to provide recommendations to caregivers or to make referrals for appropriate services. To this end, feeding is one of the most common concerns that caregivers raise during well-child visits,[64] making pediatricians the professional from whom caregivers most likely seek guidance first. One goal of this article, therefore, is to describe the characteristics of and the current state of evidence-based practices for pediatric feeding disorders to assist the pediatrician in providing anticipatory guidance. After all, one goal of pediatric prevention is to support a child's ability to thrive and remain healthy into adulthood,[65,66] and evidence-based early intervention for feeding problems is one way to do this.

Common behavioral strategies such as direct observation of behavior, consistent application of intervention, and systematic assessment of intervention efficacy are useful tools that pediatricians can recommend to caregivers. In some cases, pediatricians may need to refer children with severe feeding disorders to an intensive feeding program that provides goal-oriented, data-based assessment and intervention. Importantly, the program should incorporate interventions based on applied behavior analysis, which is the approach with the most empirical support.[15,37,67,68]

Pediatricians and behavior analysts should communicate about referrals to promote coordinated care of the child. For example, the behavior analyst should explain his or her assessment and intervention approach to ensure the pediatrician has a reasonable understanding of the planned course and can determine whether it is medically appropriate and safe. Ongoing communication during assessment and intervention is critical for assuring the child's ongoing medical care and safety. Evidently, service delivery for children with feeding disorders is an area in need of additional research to delineate the types of partnerships that will improve timely access to evidence-based services. Relatedly, future research is needed to determine how early referral and intervention for well-defined groups of children who exhibit certain risk factors (eg, failure to grow appropriately, dependence on a developmentally inappropriate source of nutrition) contributes to prevention of persistent feeding disorders.

DISCLOSURE

The authors have nothing to disclose.

REFERENCES

1. Freedman DS, Dietz WH, Srinivasan SR, et al. The relation of overweight to cardiovascular risk factors among children and adolescents: the Bogalusa Heart Study. Pediatrics 1999;103(6 Pt 1):1175–82.
2. Schreck KA, Williams K, Smith AF. A comparison of eating behaviors between children with and without autism. JAutism DevDisord 2004;34(4):433–8.
3. Ludwig DS, Majzoub JA, Al-Zahrani A, et al. High glycemic index foods, overeating, and obesity. Pediatrics 1999;103(3):E26–32.

4. Franklin L, Rodger S. Parents' perspectives on feeding medically compromised children: Implications for occupational therapy. AustOccupTher J 2003;50:137.

5. Pridham KF, Limbo R, Schroeder MM. Guided participation and development of care-giving competencies for families of low birth-weight infants. Journal of Advanced Nursing 1998;28(5):948–58.

6. Swift MC, Scholten I. Not feeding, not coming home: parental experiences of infant feeding difficulties and family relationships in a neonatal unit. J ClinNurs 2010;19(1–2):249–58.

7. Webber E, Benedict J. Postpartum depression: a multi-disciplinary approach to screening, management and breastfeeding support. Arch PsychiatrNurs 2019; 33(3):284–9.

8. Winick M, Rosso P. Head circumference and cellular growth of the brain in normal and marasmic children. JPediatr 1969;74(5):774.

9. Manikam R, Perman JA. Pediatric feeding disorders. J ClinGastroenterol 2000; 30(1):34.

10. Carruth BR, Skinner J, Houck K, et al. The phenomenon of "picky eater": a behavioral marker in eating patterns of toddlers. J Am CollNutr 1998;17(2):180–6.

11. Rommel N, De Meyer A-M, Feenstra L, et al. The complexity of feeding problems in 700 infants and young children presenting to a tertiary care institution. JPediatr-GastroenterolNutr 2003;37(1):75–84.

12. Esparo G, Canals J, Jane C, et al. Feeding problems in nursery children: Prevalence and psychosocial factors. ActaPaediatr 2004;93:663–8.

13. Chatoor I. Feeding disorders in infants and toddlers: diagnosis and intervention. Child AdolescPsychiatrClincs N Am 2002;11:163.

14. Kerwin M. Empirically supported interventions in pediatric psychology: severe feeding problems. J Pediatr Psychol 1999;24(3):193–214.

15. Volkert VM, Piazza CC. Pediatric feeding disorders. In: Sturmey P, Hersen M, editors. Handbook of evidence-based practice in clinical psychology, vol1: child and adolescent disorders. Hoboken (NJ): John Wiley & Sons Inc; 2012. p. 323–38.

16. Milnes SM, Piazza CC. Feeding disorders. In: Hastings R, Rojahn J, editors. Challenging behavior. Waltham (MA): Academic Press; 2013. p. 143–66.

17. Blackman JA, Nelson CLA. Rapid introduction of oral feedings to tube-fed patients. J DevBehavPediatr 1987;8(2):63–7.

18. Hoogewerf M, Ter Horst HJ, Groen H, et al. The prevalence of feeding problems in children formerly treated in a neonatal intensive care unit. JPerinatol 2017; 37(5):578–84.

19. Peterson KM, Ibañez VF, Kirkwood CA, et al. Assessment of pediatric feeding disorders. In: Matson JL, editor. Handbook of childhood psychopathology and developmental disabilities assessment. Springer International Publishing; 2018. p. 415–31.

20. Kerzner B, Milano K, MacLean WC Jr, et al. A practical approach to classifying and managing feeding difficulties. Pediatrics 2015;135(2):344.

21. Piazza CC. Feeding disorders and behavior: what have we learned? DevDisabil Res Rev 2008;14(2):174–81.

22. Arvedson JC, Brodsky L. Pediatric swallowing and feeding. 2nd edition. Clifton Park (NY): Delmar Cengage Learning; 2002.

23. Milnes SM, Piazza CC, Ibañez VF, et al. A comparison of Nuk presentation and Nuk redistribution to treat packing. J ApplBehav Anal 2019;52:476–90.

24. Winstock A. Eating and drinking difficulties in children. Routledge; 2017.

25. Dahlen HG, Foster JP, Psaila K, et al. Gastro-oesophageal reflux: a mixed methods study of infants admitted to hospital in the first 12 months following birth in NSW (2000–2011). BMC Pediatr 2018;18(1):1–15.

26. Rosen R, Vandenplas Y, Singendonk M, et al. Pediatric gastroesophageal reflux clinical practice guidelines. JPediatrGastroenterolNutr 2018;66(3):516–54.

27. Borowitz KC, Borowitz SM. Feeding problems in infants and children: assessment and etiology. PediatrClin North Am 2018;65(1):59–72.

28. Budd KS, McGraw TE, Farbisz R, et al. Psychosocial concomitants of children's feeding disorders. J Pediatr Psychol 1992;17(1):81–94.

29. Greer AJ, Gulotta CS, Masler EA, et al. Caregiver stress and outcomes of children with pediatric feeding disorders treated in an intensive interdisciplinary program. J Pediatr Psychol 2008;33(6):612–20.

30. Nelson SP, Chen EH, Syniar GM, et al. One-year follow-up of symptoms of gastro-esophageal reflux during infancy. Pediatrics 1998;102(6):e67.

31. Ibañez VF, Piazza CC, Peterson KM. A translational evaluation of renewal of inappropriate mealtime behavior. J ApplBehav Anal 2019;52(4):1005–20.

32. Piazza CC, Fisher WW, Brown KA, et al. Functional analysis of inappropriate mealtime behaviors. J ApplBehav Anal 2003;36:187–204.

33. Bachmeyer MH, Piazza CC, Frederick LD, et al. Functional analysis and intervention of multiply controlled inappropriate mealtime behavior. J ApplBehav Anal 2009;42:641–58.

34. Borrero CSW, Woods JN, Borrero JC, et al. Descriptive analyses of pediatric food refusal and acceptance. J ApplBehav Anal 2010;43:71–81.

35. Sharp WG, Volkert VM, Scahill L, et al. A systematic review and meta-analysis of intensive multidisciplinary intervention for pediatric feeding disorders: how standard is the standard of care? J Pediatr 2016;181:116–24.e4.

36. Sharp WG, Stubbs KH, Adams H, et al. Intensive, manual-based intervention for pediatric feeding disorders: results from a randomized pilot trial. J PediatrGastroenterolNutr 2016;62(4):658–63.

37. Laud RB, Girolami PA, Boscoe JH, et al. Intervention outcomes for severe feeding problems in children with autism spectrum disorder. BehavModif 2009;33(5):520–36.

38. Kazdin AE. Single-case research designs: methods for clinical and applied settings. Oxford University Press; 2011.

39. About the USDA Center for Nutrition Policy & Promotion. Available at: https://www.choosemyplate.gov/about-us. Accessed January 9, 2020.

40. Kerwin ME, Ahearn WH, Eicher PS, et al. The costs of eating: a behavioral economic analysis of food refusal. J ApplBehav Anal 1995;28:245–60.

41. Mueller MM, Piazza CC, Moore JW, et al. Training parents to implement pediatric feeding protocols. J ApplBehav Anal 2003;36:545–62.

42. Treloar DM. The effect of nonnutritive sucking on oxygenation in healthy, crying full-term infants. ApplNurs Res 1994;7(2):52.

43. Soxman JA. Non-nutritive sucking with a pacifier: pros and cons. Gen Dentistry 2007;55(1):59.

44. Rivas KD, Piazza CC, Kadey HJ, et al. Sequential intervention of a feeding problem using a pacifier and flipped spoon. JApplBehavAnal 2011;44:387–91.

45. Jaafar SH, Jahanfar S, Angolkar M, et al. Pacifier use versus no pacifier use in breastfeeding term infants for increasing duration of breastfeeding (review). Cochrane Database Syst Rev 2011;(3):CD007202.

46. Howard CR, Howard FM, Lanphear B, et al. Randomized clinical trial of pacifier use and bottle-feeding or cupfeeding and their effect on breastfeeding. Pediatrics 2003;111(3):511.

47. Chorna OD, Slaughter JC, Wang L, et al. A pacifier-activated music player with mother's voice improves oral feeding in preterm infants. Pediatrics 2014;133(3):462–8.
48. Pinelli J, Symington A. Non-nutritive sucking for promoting physiologic stability and nutrition in preterm infants. Cochrane Database Syst Rev 2005;(4):CD001071.
49. Ibañez VF, Kirkwood CA, Zeleny JR, et al.A pilot study on increasing intake and sucking for infants receiving supplemental feedings.BehavDev Bull, in press.
50. DeMauro SB, Abbasi S, Lorch S. The impact of feeding interval on feeding outcomes in very low birth-weight infants. J Perinatology 2011;31:481–6.
51. Lau C, Schanler RJ. Oral feeding in premature infants: advantage of a self-paced milk flow. ActaPaediatr 2000;89:453.
52. Stubbs KH, Volkert VM, Rubio EK, et al. A comparison of flipped-spoon presentation and redistribution to decrease packing in children with feeding disorders. Learn Motiv 2017;62:103–11.
53. Sharp WG, Harker S, Jaquess DL. Comparison of bite-presentation methods in the intervention of food refusal. JApplBehavAnal 2010;43:739–43.
54. Dempsey J, Piazza CC, Groff RA, et al. A flipped spoon and chin prompt to increase mouth clean. JApplBehavAnal 2011;44:961–5.
55. Volkert VM, Vaz PCM, Piazza CC, et al. Using a flipped spoon to decrease packing in children with feeding disorders. J ApplBehav Anal 2011;44:617–21.
56. Sharp WG, Odom A, Jaquess DL. Comparison of upright and flipped spoon presentations to guide intervention of food refusal. JApplBehavAnal 2012;45:83–96.
57. Wilkins JW, Piazza CC, Groff RA, et al. Chin prompt plus re-presentation as intervention for expulsion in children with feeding disorders. JApplBehavAnal 2011; 44:513–22.
58. Shalev RA, Milnes SM, Piazza CC, et al. Treating liquid expulsion in children with feeding disorders. JApplBehavAnal 2018;51:70–9.
59. Patel MR, Piazza CC, Layer SA, et al. A systematic evaluation of food textures to decrease packing and increase oral intake in children with pediatric feeding disorders. JApplBehavAnal 2005;38:89–100.
60. Zeleny JR, Volkert VM, Ibañez VF, et al. Food preferences before and during intervention for a pediatric feeding disorder. J ApplBehavAnal 2020;53:875–88.
61. Birch LL, Marlin DW. I don't like it; I never tried it: effects of exposure on two-year-old children's food preferences. Appetite 1982;3(4):353–60.
62. Cohen SA, Piazza CC, Navathe A. Feeding and nutrition. In: Crocker AC, Rubin IL, editors. Medical care for children and adults with developmental disabilities. Baltimore (MD): Paul H. Brooks; 2006. p. 295.
63. Williams KE, Riegel K, Gibbons B, et al. Intensive behavioral intervention for severe feeding problems: a cost-effective alternative to tube feeding? J DevPhysDisabil 2007;19(3):227–35.
64. Krantz J, Gievers L, Khaki S. Investigating parental concerns at the first well-child visit. ClinPediatr 2020;59(1):83–6.
65. Stanton BF. Pediatric prevention. PediatrClin North Am 2015;62(5):xv–xvi.
66. Willis E. Preventive pediatrics issues for child health care providers. PediatrClin North Am 2015;62(5):xvii–xviii.
67. Ledford JR, Gast DL. Feeding problems in children with autism spectrum disorders: a review. Focus Autism Other DevDisabl 2006;21(3):153.
68. Sharp WG, Jaquess DL, Morton JF, et al. Pediatric feeding disorders: a quantitative synthesis of intervention outcomes. Clin Child FamPsychol Rev 2010;13(4):348–65.

Pediatric Prevention
Academic Behavior

Brian K. Martens, PhD*, Emily L. Baxter, MA

KEYWORDS

- Academic problems • Response-to-intervention • Systematic formative evaluation
- Fluency • Strength of responding • Homework

KEY POINTS

- A large number of children in the United States are performing below basic standards in reading, mathematics, and writing.
- Many academic behavior problems can be traced back to deficits in basic academic skills.
- School-wide response-to-intervention models attempt to prevent academic behavior problems through universal screening, a tiered system of increasingly intensive instructional intervention, and systematic formative evaluation of child outcomes.
- The goal of school-based instructional intervention is to increase a child's strength of responding in basic academic areas so component skills can be applied to more complex composite tasks.
- Parents and caregivers can support intervention efforts at school by providing quantitative and qualitative supports for academic work completion at home.

The National Center for Education Statistics (NCES) reports on the current state of education in the United States by assessing children's performance in a variety of academic content areas. The most recent data indicate that for fourth graders across the United States, 18% are performing below basic standards in mathematics and 31% are performing below basic standards in reading.[1] That is, about 1 in 5 children in mathematics and 1 in 3 children in reading do not demonstrate even a partial understanding of content expected at their grade level. These statistics shine a spotlight on the importance of addressing academic behaviors to improve widespread deficits in children across the country.

The NCES report broadly provides evidence of the academic issues that many school districts are experiencing, but there are more specific markers that indicate academic behavior problems on a school-to-school basis. In the broadest sense, when children are not performing well on assessments such as those reported by

Department of Psychology, Syracuse University, 430 Huntington Hall, Syracuse, NY 13244-2340, USA
* Corresponding author.
E-mail address: bkmarten@syr.edu

Pediatr Clin N Am 67 (2020) 469–479
https://doi.org/10.1016/j.pcl.2020.02.002
0031-3955/20/© 2020 Elsevier Inc. All rights reserved.

the NCES, schools may see an increase in academic failure and/or rates of high-incidence disabilities. This is evidenced by students falling behind in their academics compared with same-grade peers, failing individual classes or subjects, or failing entire grades.

There are several high-incidence disabilities and diagnoses that can impact the likelihood of a child being identified as at risk for academic failure. Specific learning disabilities,[2,3] intellectual disability,[4] or emotional and behavior disorders[5] are some examples of high-incidence disabilities that children may receive diagnoses that coincide with at-risk academic performance. Although there are features of these diagnoses that may increase children's risk of academic performance deficits, academic failure is not inevitable with these diagnoses and there are evidence-based interventions that can be used to improve children's performance. It is important, however, to be aware of the increased risk inherent in these populations and include these students in universal screening procedures to identify academic behavior problems.

Identifying children who are at risk for academic problems is crucial, as academic failure is associated with several comorbid behavior problems that have implications throughout the child's life. When a child struggles with academics, he or she may engage in escape-motivated problem behavior to get out of having to complete their work,[6] such as engaging in off-task behavior (eg, sleeping, talking to other students), disrupting the teacher or class, and/or aggressing toward teachers or peers. When children engage in these challenging behaviors, they are more likely to be sent to the principal's office or in-school suspension (removal from the classroom) or even be suspended/expelled from school (removal from the school), and therefore escape the work assigned to them. These escape-motivated behaviors in turn can lead to poor peer relationships,[7] attendance problems and truancy,[8] and potentially even drop out.

SCHOOL-WIDE ACADEMIC SUPPORT SYSTEMS
Response-to-Intervention

As practitioners, we want to prevent children from falling behind or failing in their academics. There are several steps that can be taken to aid in this process. The first step is early identification of children who are struggling academically. Universal screening is a technique that schools and school districts use to identify at-risk students. This screening process is typically nested within a response-to-intervention (RtI) tiered support system,[9] and involves student support teams administering curriculum-based measurement (CBM) probes in the basic areas of mathematics, reading, and writing. These probes are brief (1–3 minute) samples of child performance on curriculumlike materials (eg, reading a 150-word passage, working math computation problems) that are scored for accurate rate (eg, words read correctly per minute [WRCM]). By administering CBM probes at fall, winter, and spring benchmarking periods, schools can track the progress of all students, identify children who are performing below the level of same-grade peers, and identify children whose rate of improvement is below that of their peers between assessments.[10] Both classroom teachers and parents may also refer children directly to their school's pupil service team for possible instructional intervention and more frequent progress monitoring. *Systematic formative evaluation* involves the use of CBM probes to more frequently monitor children's academic progress and graph session-by-session performance data.[11] This practice allows teachers to determine exactly when to change instructional goals and methods by either (1) moving forward to a more demanding goal or using more difficult instructional materials when a goal is met, or (2) moving backward to a less demanding goal or using less difficult instructional materials if the child shows little or no improvement over time. In their meta-analysis of the effects of systematic formative evaluation on student performance, Fuchs and Fuchs[11] found that teachers who engaged in systematic formative evaluation made more frequent instructional changes, which resulted in an average effect size of 0.70 on student achievement.

Level of performance and rate of improvement across assessment times are 2 major considerations when deciding whether intervention is needed for a child's academic performance. Known as a *dual-discrepancy criterion*,[9] when a child is performing at levels well below their peers, and their rate of improvement under current instruction or intervention is not sufficient to bring performance levels up to that of their peers, the child is identified as at risk for academic failure. Schools that use RtI for identifying and intervening early with students who are at risk for academic failure will generally use a 3-tier intervention system[12]:

- *Tier 1 (primary prevention).* This is the general education curriculum to which all students have access. Universal screening is typically completed at fall, winter, and spring benchmarking periods to identify at-risk children.
- *Tier 2 (secondary prevention).* Children who are not responding to the general education curriculum receive more intensive small-group instruction using a standard protocol intervention. Progress is monitored frequently (1–2 times weekly) using systematic formative evaluation to determine if intervention should be continued, scaled back, or if additional services are needed.
- *Tier 3 (tertiary prevention).* In this tier, children who continue to perform at a lower level than their peers and do not demonstrate sufficient growth receive individualized education programming. If there is no response to intervention in this tier, a psychoeducational evaluation is conducted to determine the child's eligibility for classification and placement as a child with a disability.

As systematic formative evaluation is completed within this RtI system, children who are identified as having a dual discrepancy in both level and rate of improvement in their performance are provided a more intensive intervention (ie, at tier 2 or tier 3). If their academic performance improves, then the academic support team within the school will determine if their services should be continued as a supplement to regular instruction or scaled back.

School-Wide Positive Behavior Support

Due to the escape-motivated problem behavior that often co-occurs with at-risk academic performance (ie, children who engage in disruptive behavior to avoid or get out of schoolwork), schools generally will have a parallel tiered system in place to intervene early with challenging classroom behavior. Known as a school-wide positive behavior support system, reinforcement programs are put in place to increase positive behaviors within the classroom.[13] These behavior supports also work in a tiered system like RtI to ensure that all levels of need are covered. Tier 1 or universal positive behavior supports are offered or provided to the entire school for a specific behavior that is being targeted.[12] For example, if the school is trying to increase daily attendance, the administrative team could provide a pizza day at lunch for the classroom that has the most children with perfect attendance over a specific period of time.

For behaviors that require additional or higher intensity intervention, more personalized reinforcement programs for on-task and/or desired classroom behavior are used. Teaching children how to appropriately ask for a break or providing breaks for increasingly longer durations of on-task behavior are 2 techniques that can be used to decrease escape-motivated problem behavior and increase task completion.

Tier 1 or universal interventions for both academic and behavioral needs require relatively less effort from school administration, faculty, and staff to implement. Implementing more intensive and personalized instructional or behavioral interventions at Tiers 2 and 3, however, requires additional effort to create plans and train staff to implement these plans with high levels of treatment fidelity.

Student Support and Intervention Teams

Within most school districts and individual schools, there are staff members who make up what is sometimes called a student intervention team (SIT).[13] SITs are made up of school psychologists, social workers, teachers, and administrators, and occasionally the child will also be involved in goal setting for themselves. Individuals who are part of SIT will review progress data for at-risk student(s) to determine the next steps in intervention. This team will set goals for data collection by operationalizing the specific behavior change(s) they want for each child. This can include both increasing performance in a specific academic area (eg, math or reading) and/or decreasing problem behavior within the classroom. SITs typically meet at least once per week, review CBM probe or behavior observation data that have been collected, determine the next course of action, and set goals for the following meeting. Goals may include recording data on a new area of concern or reviewing improvement in a previously discussed area.

Within schools, the SIT is crucial in ensuring that appropriate evidence-based interventions are chosen for each at-risk student and that data are collected to monitor progress. In the following section, the key principles, strategies, and tactics of instructional interventions used by SITs are discussed.

FUNDAMENTALS OF INSTRUCTIONAL INTERVENTION
Component Versus Composite Skills

In schools, the academic skills taught, the sequence in which they are taught, and the instructional materials used are dictated by a curriculum. In a typical curriculum sequence, basic skill areas are linked within grade levels and increase in difficulty across grade levels. In reading, for example, children in first grade are expected to learn phonological awareness, phonics and decoding, and sight-word vocabulary skills.[14] Phonological awareness tasks might involve showing children index cards containing sound segments of words separated by lines (eg, c/l/aw) and having them blend the sounds to make a word.[15] For sight-word training, children might be shown lists of words and told to say each word in its entirety after modeling by the teacher.

In grades 2 and 3, the focus of reading instruction shifts to fluent reading of connected text and reading comprehension.[14] These tasks require children to apply previously learned phonological awareness, decoding, and vocabulary skills to quickly read and understand stories and passages. Teaching these more advanced skills requires giving children short stories to practice and comprehension questions to answer.

At higher grades, children are expected to smoothly coordinate a number of basic skills to respond quickly and accurately to complex academic tasks (eg, preparing a book report in middle school). As noted earlier, performing below same-grade peers on more complex tasks like classroom activities and teacher-made tests, district-wide reading, math, and writing assessments, or universal CBM screening probes are important markers of academic behavior problems.

Many academic behavior problems can be traced back to deficits in basic academic skills. These basic or *component skills* can be thought of as the building blocks for more complex, *composite skills*.[16,17] For example, subtraction with borrowing and multiplication are component skills for long division. Children who have not yet learned or are slow at performing these component skills will have difficulty learning long division, placing them at risk for academic behavior problems. More generally, as children encounter increasingly more difficult curricular demands, deficits in component skills can accumulate to slow down or even prevent the learning of complex, composite skills.[18]

Strength of Responding

An important concept in children's ability to combine or apply component skills to solve more complex tasks is *strength of responding*.[19] Strength of responding refers to how proficient a child is at performing the skill or set of skills being taught. Mastery does not occur all at once. Rather, strength of responding increases gradually along a continuum as children are given more opportunities to practice a skill with modeling, prompting, reinforcement, and feedback. For children who are first learning a new skill, responding is often tenuous and fraught with errors. The goal for children at this level is to perform the skill correctly on most or all training trials (ie, accuracy). Achieving this goal indicates that the child has met the minimum criterion for initially "learning" the new skill. Once a child can perform the skill accurately, the next goal is to perform it accurately and quickly when responding to strings of item while being timed (ie, fluency). Some experts suggest that 70% of instructional time should be devoted to fluency building,[20] and the National Reading Panel concluded that fluency in basic skills like oral reading and decoding is essential for reading comprehension.[21] When skills can be performed accurately and quickly during instruction, the final goal is to apply the skill accurately and quickly to solve complex tasks outside of training (ie, generalization). Children's ability to generalize skills to untrained material has been shown to increase with strength of responding and the similarity of that material to what was trained.[15,18,22]

Research suggests that attempts to train more complex aspects of responding (eg, generalization) may not succeed until children achieve more basic accuracy and/or fluency goals.[18,23] Conversely, prolonged practice beyond an initial accuracy criterion (ie, overlearning or fluency training) has been shown to promote generalization, increase retention in the absence of practice, and increase endurance over longer work intervals.[15,24–26] Strength of responding is also important because different instructional methods have been shown to better promote learning at different proficiency levels.[16] Instructional methods refer to how opportunities for the child to respond are structured during an intervention session, the type of help a teacher or parent gives *before* the child responds, and how often adults reinforce correct responses and correct errors *after* the child responds.

Acquisition-level training

Opportunities to respond during an intervention session can be structured either as discrete trials by presenting one stimulus (eg, a sight-word) at a time and giving the child a single, discrete opportunity to respond, or by presenting strings of stimuli (eg, a 150-word story) to which the child can respond freely (ie, a free-operant format). A discrete-trial format is generally recommended for acquisition-level training because it allows SIT members to model, prompt, and correct errors for each child response, which in turn decreases errors and escape-motivated problem behavior. For discrete-trial sessions, training goals are typically stated as the percentage of correct trials performed independently (without modeling or prompting) over some desired number of consecutive sessions (eg, 90% correct independent trials over 3 consecutive sessions). During acquisition-level training, help is provided before a child responds in the form of modeling, prompting, or strategy instruction. Modeling involves demonstrating a correct response for the child, whereas prompting involves SIT members pointing to, partially telling, or guiding a correct response. For more complex tasks, strategy instruction involves describing each skill in a sequence, modeling application of the skill using a "think aloud" strategy, and allowing the child to practice the skill on their own.[27] During acquisition-level training, reinforcement of correct responses and correction of errors are critical for teaching what response is expected to the stimulus materials presented.

Fluency-level training

A free-operant format is required for fluency training because accurate rate of responding rather than percentage of accurate responses is measured. Fluency goals are stated as the correct number of responses during a brief interval (eg, 100 WRCM in reading, 45 digits correct per minute in math computation). Normative fluency standards in reading, math, and writing are available (eg, DIBELS and AIMSweb[28]), and SITs should consult these when setting fluency training goals. When practicing to build fluency, the expectation is that children will respond correctly to most or all of the items presented. As such, help provided during acquisition-level training is withdrawn and replaced with brief, repeated practice opportunities on material that is, matched to the child's proficiency level. When the fluency goal is met on one set of material, the difficulty level is increased and practice continues. Reinforcement during fluency training is contingent on both speed and accuracy, and may involve goal setting, performance charting, praise, or tokens exchangeable for preferred items.[26]

Generalization-level training

Promoting the application of skills trained in one set of conditions to other, untrained conditions is arguably the goal of all academic instruction. Intervening to promote this level of proficiency requires that the stimuli used in training be diversified or selected in such a way as to be representative of the generalization context. For example, a variety of strategies have been examined for promoting generalized oral reading fluency and include training loosely with multiple passages, training with passages containing multiple exemplars of key words, onsets, or rimes, training to functional fluency aims (eg, at least 100 WRCM), and training broadly applicable skills like rapid phoneme blending.[15,22,29–31]

Selecting Evidence-Based Instructional Interventions

Once a child has been identified as at risk for academic failure and in need of tier 2 or 3 supports, SIT members must select an evidence-based instructional intervention that is matched to the child's proficiency level. This means pinpointing the type of deficit the child is exhibiting and then selecting an intervention that is appropriate for the child's level of proficiency that can be implemented as often as is practical in the child's regular education classroom, and that can be implemented with fidelity.

Daly and colleagues[32] described 5 reasons for academic behavior deficits based on a child's instructional history. These 5 reasons map onto acquisition-level, fluency-level, and generalization-level goals and therefore can be used by SITs to select instructional interventions:

- *"They don't want to do it"* because academic responding has not been sufficiently reinforced in the past to make it enjoyable. In such cases, intervention consisting of a structured reinforcement program (ie, providing incentives) may be sufficient to strengthen responding. SIT members can determine if simple reinforcement or additional instruction involving modeling, prompting, error correction, or practice is needed by conducting a performance-deficit analysis (PDA).[33] In a PDA, various intervention components (eg, reinforcement, modeling via passage previewing, practice via repeated readings) are applied to equivalent but different stimulus materials and the child's response to each component is measured. Whatever component (or combination of components) is shown to improve performance the most is then implemented over time as a Tier 2 or 3 intervention.
- *"It's too hard,"* meaning that the instructional materials are too difficult for the child's skill level. In such cases, slicing back by allowing the child to practice the same skills on less difficult material may strengthen responding.
- *"They haven't had enough help to do it,"* meaning they have not received enough modeling, prompting, or strategy instruction to establish accurate performance of the skill. In this case, additional, intensive instruction is required.
- *"They haven't spent enough time doing it"* or have not practiced the skill long enough to build fluency or promote retention, endurance, and generalization. Here, brief, repeated practice opportunities with goal setting and reinforcement are required to build fluency.
- *"They haven't done it that way before"* meaning that instruction ended before children were given varied opportunities to apply the skill in situations different from training. In such cases, SIT members can probe for generalization on materials different from those used in training (ie, CBM global outcome measures) and either continue to build fluency until generalization is observed or systematically diversify the training materials.[22]

INSTRUCTIONAL SUPPORTS AT HOME

Although much progress can be made with interventions implemented at school for students who are at risk for academic failure, children spend only approximately 25% to 30% of their time at school.[34] Therefore, it is important to consider how parents and caregivers can support children's academic progress at home where they spend most of their time.

School/Caregiver Relationship-Building Techniques

One of the first steps a parent or caregiver can take in supporting their child's academic progress at home is building a connection with their child's school. This can be done in a general sense (eg, joining the school's parent-teacher organization or volunteering in the classroom), but also on an individual level by building relationships with the faculty and staff who interact with their child.

In the school-caregiver research literature, these connections are known as family-school partnerships. Family-school partnerships have been shown to improve student outcomes, such as academic achievement.[35] The National Center for School Engagement (NCSE) provided recommendations for effective family-school partnerships based on the Epstein Method of family-school partnerships.[36,37] These recommendations include the following:

- *Creating consistent 2-way communication between the family and the school.* This is especially crucial when a child is at risk for academic failure. The family should be kept informed about what is occurring at school regarding SIT considerations and child progress, and the school should be informed of any outside interventions occurring (eg, applied behavior analysis, occupational, or physical therapy) and any progress that has been noted at home.

- *Being involved in school decision-making processes.* Parent involvement with school decision making can occur on a larger systems level (eg, participating in committees within the school) or on an individual level involving their child. Parents of children who are at risk for academic failure should be kept informed of any interventions currently in place and remain involved in any decision making that is directly related to their child's intervention and progress.
- *Creating an effective and structured learning environment at home.* The NCSE recommends 3 activities a parent or caregiver can engage in to provide instructional support at home. These include helping the child organize their time (eg, limiting screen time and making a homework routine), assisting the child with homework when needed, and opening communication channels with their child about short-term and long-term educational goals.

General Homework Support Recommendations

Parental involvement in homework assignments and tasks has been shown to improve academic achievement, and there are different types of involvement that can lead to these outcomes.[35] The 2 main ways that parents and caregivers can assist with homework have been labeled as *quantitative* and *qualitative support*. Quantitative supports include activities such as actually completing the homework with the child (eg, working problems together, modeling and prompting to elicit a correct response, correcting errors). Qualitative supports are activities that ensure an effective learning environment like setting rules for homework completion or removing distractions in the environment.

The National Association of School Psychologists (NASP) provided guidelines for parents that align with quantitative and qualitative supports for successful homework completion.[38] These guidelines include parents or caregivers

- Checking with their child each day after school to review any homework assignments that have been given.
- Creating a consistent homework routine. For example, each night after dinner the child will complete any homework from school (or practice skills if no homework has been assigned) for 30 minutes before engaging in any screen time or receiving dessert.
- Providing supervision as children complete their homework in the least intrusive way possible. That is, parents and caregivers should ensure that children are completing their work and provide quantitative assistance as needed, but not so much assistance that the child becomes dependent on parental feedback and help. It is recommended to use least-to-most prompting (ie, use a less intrusive prompt and increase help as necessary to elicit a correct response) to ensure autonomy and independence in work completion.
- Enlisting siblings or peers to help children with homework completion. This takes some of the pressure off the parent, allows additional practice for the sibling/peer, and gives the child a different perspective on work completion.
- Providing explicit, programmed reinforcement or incentives for homework completion when necessary. For example, using "first, then" statements can be effective in increasing motivation to finish homework efficiently and accurately, such as "first, complete 10 minutes of math problems, then you can play games on the tablet for 5 minutes."

A SUMMARY OF BEST PRACTICES IN PREVENTING ACADEMIC BEHAVIOR PROBLEMS

Based on the structure of school-wide academic support systems, the fundamentals of instructional intervention, and NASP guidelines for supporting homework completion, we conclude with a list of "best practice" recommendations for preventing academic behavior problems:

- Screen all children for basic skill deficits using CBM global outcome measures.
- Provide a tier-2 standard protocol intervention for children who are at risk for academic failure at this stage.
- Engage in frequent home-school communication to involve parents and caregivers in SIT decision making and to create an effective and structured learning environment at home.
- Monitor the child's progress at least twice weekly on the material being instructed as well as on CBM global outcome measures to probe for generalization and graph the data (ie, systematic formative evaluation).
- Evaluate progress using a dual-discrepancy criterion. Is the child below same-grade peers in both level and slope of improvement?
- Provide a tier-3 individualized intervention for children who are at risk for academic failure at this stage.
- Conduct a PDA to rule out "Won't do" versus "Can't do" problems and identify strength of responding in the targeted content area based on the 5 reasons for academic behavior problems.
- Implement an evidence-based intervention matched to the child's proficiency level (ie, to strengthen accuracy, fluency, or generalization) and continue to monitor progress.
- Provide qualitative support for academics at home by creating a consistent homework routine using "first, then" statements, setting goals for homework completion, creating a homework environment free of distractions, and reinforcing homework completion consistent with the "first-then" statements.
- Provide quantitative support for academics at home by helping the child with assigned work using modeling, least-to-most prompting, error correction, and reinforcement for correct responses.

DISCLOSURE

The authors have nothing to disclose.

REFERENCES

1. National Center for Educational Statistics. How did U.S. students perform on the most recent assessments?. 2017. Available at: http://www.nationsreportcard.gov. Accessed June 22, 2019.
2. McLean JF, Hitch GJ. Working memory impairments in children with specific arithmetic learning difficulties. J Exp Child Psychol 1999;74:240–60.
3. Lewis C, Hitch GJ, Walker P. The prevalence of specific arithmetic difficulties and specific reading difficulties in 9- to 10-year-old boys and girls. J Child Psychol Psychiatry 1994;35:283–92.
4. Sabornie EJ, Cullinan D, Osborne SS, et al. Intellectual, academic, and behavioral functioning of students with high-incidence disabilities: a cross-categorical meta-analysis. Exceptional Children 2005;72:47–63.

5. Lane KL, Wehby J, Barton-Arwood SM. Students with and at risk for emotional and behavioral disorders: meeting their social and academic needs. Preventing School Failure 2005;49(2):6–9.

6. Beavers GA, Iwata BA, Lerman DC. Thirty years of research on the functional analysis of problem behavior. J Appl Behav Anal 2013;46:1–21.

7. Dishion TJ, Patterson GR, Stoolmiller M, et al. Family, school, and behavioral antecedents to early adolescent involvement with antisocial peers. Dev Psychol 1991;27(1):172–80.

8. Berg I. School refusal and truancy. Arch Dis Child 1997;76:90–1.

9. Hughes CA, Dexter DD. Response to intervention: a research-based summary. Theory Pract 2011;50:4–11.

10. Good RH, Simmons DC, Kame'enui EJ. The importance and decision-making utility of a continuum of fluency-based indicators of foundational reading skills for third-grade high-stakes outcomes. Sci Stud Read 2001;5:257–88.

11. Fuchs LS, Fuchs D. Effects of systematic formative evaluation: a meta-analysis. Except Child 1986;53:199–208.

12. Fuchs LS, Fuchs D. A model for implementing responsiveness to intervention. Teaching Exceptional Children 2007;39(5):14–20.

13. Burns MK, Symington T. A meta-analysis of prereferral intervention teams: student and systemic outcomes. J Sch Psychol 2002;40:437–47.

14. Snow CE, Burns SM, Griffin P, editors. Preventing reading difficulties in young children. Washington, DC: National Academy Press; 1998.

15. Martens BK, Werder CS, Hier BO, et al. Fluency training in phoneme blending: a preliminary study of generalized effects. J Behav Educ 2013;22:16–36.

16. Martens BK, Codding RS, Sallade SJ. School-based instructional support. In: Luiselli JK, editor. Applied behavior analysis advanced guidebook. London: Academic Press/Elsevier; 2017. p. 167–95.

17. Lin F, Kubina R Jr. A preliminary investigation of the relationship between fluency and application for multiplication. J Behav Educ 2005;14:73–87.

18. Binder C. Behavioral fluency: evolution of a new paradigm. Behav Analyst 1996; 19:163–97.

19. Martens BK, Daly EJ, Begeny JC, et al. Behavioral approaches to education. In: Fisher W, Piazza C, Roane H, editors. Handbook of applied behavior analysis. 2nd edition. New York: Guilford; in press.

20. Johnson KR, Layng TVJ. On terms and procedures: fluency. Behav Analyst 1996; 19:281–8.

21. National Reading Panel. Teaching children to read: an evidence-based assessment of the scientific research literature on reading and its implications for reading instruction. Washington, DC: National Institutes of Health; 2000.

22. Martens BK, Young ND, Mullane MP, et al. Effects of word overlap on generalized gains from a repeated readings intervention. J Sch Psychol 2019;74:1–9.

23. Lannie AL, Martens BK. Targeting performance dimensions in sequence according to the Instructional Hierarchy: effects on children's math work within a self-monitoring program. J Behav Educ 2008;17:356–75.

24. Driskell JE, Willis RP, Copper C. Effect of overlearning on retention. J Appl Psychol 1992;77:615–22.

25. Lee GT, Singer-Dudek J. Effects of fluency versus accuracy training on endurance and retention of assembly tasks by four adolescents with developmental disabilities. J Behav Educ 2012;21:1–17.

26. Martens BK, Eckert TL, Begeny JC, et al. Effects of a fluency-building program on the reading performance of low-achieving second and third grade students. J Behav Educ 2007;16:39–54.
27. Hough TM, Hixson MD, Decker D, et al. The effectiveness of an explicit instruction writing program for second graders. J Behav Educ 2012;21:163–74.
28. Good RH, Kaminski RA. Dynamic indicators of basic early literacy skills. 5th edition. Eugene (OR): Institute for the Development of Educational Achievement; 2001. Available at: http://dibels.uoregon.edu/. Accessed February 6, 2017.
29. Ardoin SP, Binder KS, Zawoyski AM, et al. Using eye-tracking procedures to evaluate generalization effects: practicing target words during repeated readings within versus across texts. Sch Psychol Rev 2013;42:477–95.
30. Bonfiglio CM, Daly EJ, Martens BK, et al. An experimental analysis of reading interventions: generalization across instructional strategies, time, and passages. J Appl Behav Anal 2004;37:111–4.
31. Silber JM, Martens BK. Programming for the generalization of oral reading fluency: repeated readings of entire text versus multiple exemplars. J Behav Educ 2010;19:30–46.
32. Daly EJ, Witt JC, Martens BK, et al. A model for conducting a functional analysis of academic performance problems. Sch Psychol Rev 1997;26:554–74.
33. Daly EJ, Martens BK, Dool EJ, et al. Using brief functional analysis to select interventions for oral reading. J Behav Educ 1998;8:203–18.
34. Clark RN. Why disadvantaged children succeed. Public Welfare at ProQuest Central; 1990. p. 17–23.
35. Dettmers S, Yotyodying S, Jonkmann K. Antecedents and outcomes of parental homework involvement: How do family-school partnerships affect parental homework involvement and student outcomes? Front Psychol 2019;10:1–13.
36. National Center for School Engagement. What research says about family-school-community partnerships. 2005. Available at: www.schoolengagement.org. Accessed June 22, 2019.
37. Epstein JL. School, family, and community partnerships: preparing educators and improving schools. London: Taylor and Francis; 2018.
38. National Association of School Psychologists. Homework: a guide for parents. Bethesda (MD): Peg Dawson, EDD, NCSP; 2010.

Making the Most of Clinical Encounters

Prevention of Child Abuse and Maltreatment

Iram J. Ashraf, MD, Alicia R. Pekarsky, MD, JoAnne E. Race, MS,
Ann S. Botash, MD*

KEYWORDS

- Parenting • Child maltreatment • Neglect • Sexual abuse • Sentinel injuries

KEY POINTS

- Risk factors for child abuse vary depending on age, developmental factors, social context, and type of abuse.
- Support for parents is critical for prevention efforts.
- Selecting appropriate resources, based on risks and type of abuse, requires understanding of local programs.
- Recognition of physical findings, particularly sentinel injuries, is necessary to prevent further abuse.
- Sexual abuse prevention requires recognition of subtle signs, including signs of trafficking and peer victimization.

INTRODUCTION

Childhood experiences occur within the context of family and community and this context may include child abuse, maltreatment, and neglect. Child abuse is a public health concern with great costs to not only children and families, but also to society. Abused children suffer physical injuries, psychological problems, learning difficulties, a spectrum of neurologic sequelae, and death. Abused children grow up to be adults at risk for depression, suicide, substance abuse, and criminal activity and are at higher risk for abusing children themselves.[1]

Gaps in physician knowledge and skills and discomfort in addressing child maltreatment impede prevention efforts.[2] In addition, the US Preventive Services Task Force, the American Academy of Family Practitioners, and the American Academy of

State University of New York Upstate Medical University, Upstate Golisano Children's Hospital, Department of Pediatrics, 750 East Adams Street, Syracuse, NY 13210, USA
* Corresponding author.
E-mail address: BOTASHA@UPSTATE.EDU
Twitter: @Botash (A.S.B.)

Pediatr Clin N Am 67 (2020) 481–498
https://doi.org/10.1016/j.pcl.2020.02.004
0031-3955/20/© 2020 Elsevier Inc. All rights reserved.
pediatric.theclinics.com

Pediatrics (AAP) have no recommendations for primary care interventions to prevent child maltreatment. However, the US Preventive Services Task Force report notes that primary care physicians, including pediatricians and others, are uniquely positioned to identify child maltreatment.[3] The AAP strongly recommends clinician involvement in preventing child maltreatment and provides guidance and information on risk factors, protective factors, and clinical management.[2]

The authors used the three-tiered public health framework for prevention (primary, secondary, and tertiary) to guide strategies for clinical encounters.[4] In the current paper, we discuss how providers can identify, address, and prevent child maltreatment through parent education and use appropriate programs. This discussion includes a review of early intervention resources, summaries of strategies, and an overview of prevention approaches for neglect, physical abuse, head trauma, sexual abuse, and peer victimization.

PUBLIC HEALTH PREVENTION FRAMEWORK

The public health prevention framework aids in categorizing programs.

- Primary prevention programs are population-based and engage the community. These may include home visits from a nurse and/or provision of parenting information and education. Strategies focus on addressing risk factors. Primary prevention offers the best opportunity to reduce long-term sequelae of child maltreatment by preventing trauma to the developing brain during the first 3 years of life.[5]
- Secondary prevention programs target families with specific risk factors for child maltreatment.
- Tertiary prevention programs are designed to prevent maltreatment recurrence and adverse outcomes from abusive experiences.

Tertiary prevention strategies can be provided during ongoing pediatric health care for children who have been maltreated.[6] Maximizing health care and services for maltreated children after they return to their biologic homes from foster or kinship care can be offered through anticipatory guidance. Important prevention considerations for postabuse follow-up include assessment of risks for recidivism in families; close monitoring of developmental milestones, especially in children where head trauma occurred; monitoring of behavioral changes caused by family and possible cultural adjustments; and medical concerns related to the abusive injuries.[6]

IDENTIFYING RISK FACTORS FOR ABUSE AND MALTREATMENT

Parent or caregiver characteristics and psychological functioning, characteristics of the child, and the social context within which the family unit lives influence parenting methods.[7] Within these components are several risk factors for the abuse and maltreatment of children. Parental stress is a common denominator.

Poor Parenting Skills

Parents who have inadequate knowledge of normal and expected child development are at risk for demonstrating poor parenting skills and this increases the risk for maltreatment.[5,8] Parental knowledge deficits may be caused by a lack of a good parenting model, lack of previous exposure to children, the parent's own developmental delays or emotional issues, and a lack of knowledge regarding normal child development, or other reasons. For example, a parent who believes a 1 year old should be capable of understanding the consequences of touching a hot mug might leave the mug within reach of a child. Some parents believe in the success of corporal punishment and lack knowledge and skills for effective disciplinary strategies.[7] Those who use harsh, inattentive, or inconsistent parenting are at higher risk of abusing their children.[9] Parental characteristics culminating in poor parent-child relationships further increase the risk of child maltreatment.[7]

Parental Psychological Functioning

Parents with mental health concerns, such as depression, anxiety, and high levels of stress, are at risk for maltreating their children.[7] They may have difficulty adhering to appropriate parenting practices and coping with childcare.[9] Parents who abuse substances may have altered judgment and mentation caring for their child.

Risk factors, or combination of factors, that may lead to mental health concerns also increase risk for child abuse, including

- Intimate partner violence
- A parent with a history of being abused as a child[1]
- A history of other trauma
- Social issues, such as poverty and neighborhood violence

Societal Factors Affecting Parenting

Structural issues can lead to compromised functioning of parents and cause increased family stress. These may include

- Homelessness and lack of housing assistance[9]
- Living in high-poverty communities[5,8]
- Living in violent neighborhoods
- Food insecurity
- Parental social isolation[5,8]
- Limited access to services that promote parental mental and physical well-being

Difficult to Care for Children

Children with developmental and/or physical disabilities, behavioral issues, and chronic medical conditions are at increased risk for maltreatment.[9] Children with such characteristics often require higher levels of care and nurturing and are challenging for even the most experienced parent. For a parent with inadequate parenting skills or other risk factors, parenting a child with a disability may be extremely stressful.

Other Risk Factors

Children younger than 3 years of age are especially vulnerable.[5,8] One-third of children who are maltreated are between the ages of 0 and 3 years, with most victims being younger than 1 year of age.[10] An important risk includes having a nonbiologically related adult in the home, because these adults are often the perpetrators of maltreatment.[9] However, nonbiologically related adults are not always the abuser. Children may be abused by any caregiver.

ABUSIVE HEAD TRAUMA

Abusive head trauma (AHT), formerly referred to as shaken baby syndrome, describes the signs and symptoms resulting from nonaccidental shaking of the head and neck, impacting of the head and neck area, or a combination of acceleration/deceleration injury and impact.

Infant crying is a common trigger for AHT. This association is based on age-specific curves for AHT that have similar onset and patterns as age-specific curves for crying. Crying usually increases during the first month of life, peaks in the second month, and decreases by the fourth month.[11] The incidence of AHT peaks between 2.5 to 4 months, with the first episode estimated to occur around 6 weeks of age.[12,13]

Parents commonly ask primary care providers about the causes of infant crying and how to manage it.[13] An infant with prolonged and inconsolable episodes of crying is a source of anger, frustration, powerlessness, and stress.[11] These feelings may be overwhelming and lead to caregiver loss of control and violence toward the infant.[13]

Parents may not know an infant's brain is fragile or understand the consequences of shaking a baby. In one study, 25% to 50% of future parents did not know shaking a baby could lead to brain injury or death.[14] Low-cost prevention programs provided by maternity nurses before newborn discharge demonstrated promising results.[15] Later data using a larger cohort indicated that, despite retained self-reported parental knowledge, head trauma hospitalization rates were not reduced.[16]

PREVENTION STRATEGIES

Successful interventions not only reduce risk factors but also promote protective factors. Families with good social supports have lower rates of physical abuse and are more likely to use nonphysical disciplinary strategies.[9,17] A parent's sense of self-efficacy and competence enables better coping strategies and reduces the adverse effects of risk factors. For example, parents who can secure resources and services for their family's particular needs, such as services for a developmentally delayed child, are much less likely to abuse.[9,18] Similarly, children with high self-esteem who have the supportive involvement of an adult or who are involved in extracurricular activities, may be less likely to suffer the negative consequences of maltreatment.[9,19]

Education and support are important prevention strategies.[7] Some strategies may be implemented through local community resources, such as home visiting or referral to a parenting program, and others may involve direct provider-to-family interaction.

Parenting programs are one of the most successful interventions for reducing child maltreatment in those with identified risk factors.[7] Evidence has shown that parenting programs are successful in reducing the prevalence of reports of child maltreatment, preventing its recurrence, and reducing the risk factors that impair healthy functioning.[7]

Medical providers may need to develop skills in identifying risks for maltreatment and preparation for offering prevention strategies. The Safe Environment for Every Kid (SEEK) model has been reported to enable practitioners to identify and help address psychosocial problems (ie, parental depression, substance abuse, major stress, intimate partner violence, harsh punishment, and food insecurity) associated with neglect.[20] Results of randomized controlled trials have demonstrated promising outcomes regarding the efficacy of the SEEK model.[21] For example, in an urban pediatric resident clinic, SEEK resulted in significantly lower rates of child maltreatment in all outcome measures: decreased child protective services (CPS) reports, problems related to neglect, nonadherence to medical care, delayed immunizations, and rates of severe/very severe physical punishment.[1]

Selecting and Implementing Effective Prevention Resources

To offer comprehensive and useful local resources for families, providers must assess the effectiveness of local programs. Referrals may be influenced by

- The effectiveness of programs based on local funding, staffing, needs, and other concerns
- The program's theory (eg, interventions for parenting skills vs intervention for parents with mental health concerns)

- Form of abuse, such as head trauma prevention, support for families at risk for neglecting children, child sexual abuse (CSA) prevention programs, and others

The clearinghouse model is used to help evaluate effectiveness and inform decision-makers about validated evidence-based practices of prevention programs. Clearinghouses use simple formats to summarize empirical evidence supporting program efficacy. The California Evidence-Based Clearinghouse for Child Welfare (CEBC) offers a database of child welfare–related programs with a rating system, descriptions, and resources, including a guide to program selection and implementation. CEBC includes topic areas within primary and secondary prevention (**Table 1**).[22] Programs that address bullying, cyberbullying, harassment, bystander actions, consent, gender, and social norms education have the potential to reduce the public health challenge of CSA.[23]

Parenting Programs

Most home visiting and parent education programs successfully reduce child maltreatment.[7,24] Components of data-based parenting programs include attachment theory, learning theory, and social learning theory principles to change parenting attitudes, practices, skills, reduction of parent-child conflict, reduction of parenting stress, improvement of psychosocial functioning, improvement of daily dynamics, and reduction of child behavioral problems.[25] Chen and Chan[7] found that programs produced positive effects in low-, middle-, and high-income countries and were effective in reducing child maltreatment when applied as primary, secondary, and tertiary maltreatment interventions. The risk of maltreatment decreased after interventions. Fathers did not gain as much from parenting programs as mothers and programs may need modification for fathers. The authors also found that parenting programs started on or before the prenatal period were helpful in preventing maltreatment from ever occurring.[7]

Home visiting through nurse-family partnerships[24] directed toward high-risk populations, such as adolescent parents, have focused on interventions that improve neurodevelopmental, cognitive, and behavioral functioning of the child using theories of human ecology, self-efficacy, and human attachment. Nurse-family partnership programs are offered in 41 states and local resources are identified through the national Web site.[26]

The AAP has developed prevention programs for clinical settings including Connected Kids: Safe, Strong, Secure, a resiliency-based educational program for parents and providers focused on managing challenging developmental stages, providing effective discipline, and other topics. The effectiveness of this program has not yet been evaluated.[27] Practicing Safety is another AAP-developed program that helps providers screen for and address maternal depression. It uses anticipatory guidance to help parents cope with challenging developmental stages, such as infant crying, colic, and toilet training.[28] Changes in practice behavior have been demonstrated, but effects on child maltreatment have not been examined.[9]

Other prevention education may include

- Staying Positive While Parenting, a free, online resource, is available through the New York State Department Health grant-funded program for child abuse medical providers. These handouts were developed to help parents manage their own emotions when facing children's challenging developmental stages.[29]
- The Centers for Disease Control and Prevention offers further guidance regarding violence prevention on their Web site.[30]
- All child caregivers, athletic coaches, and other adults who may have independent access to children may pose risks to any child. Steps to choosing

Table 1
Programs in primary and secondary prevention of child abuse and neglect

Child Welfare Related Program	Type of Prevention	Target Audience	CEBC Rating[a]	Program Information
Nurse-Family Partnership	Primary	Home visits for first-time low-income mothers with children from pregnancy through second birthday	1; well-supported by research evidence	https://www.cebc4cw.org/program/nurse-family-partnership/
Safe Environment for Every Kid	Primary	Families with children to age 5	1; well-supported by research evidence	https://www.cebc4cw.org/program/safe-environment-for-every-kid-seek-model/
Triple P Positive Parenting Program System	Primary	For parents and caregivers of children to age 16	2; supported by research evidence	https://www.cebc4cw.org/program/triple-p-positive-parenting-program-system/
ACT Raising Safe Kids	Primary	Parents and caregivers of children birth to age 10	3; promising research	https://www.cebc4cw.org/program/act-raising-safe-kids/
"Who Do you Tell?"	Primary	Children kindergarten to grade 6	3; promising research	https://www.cebc4cw.org/program/who-do-you-tell/
Body Safety Training Workbook	Primary	Children ages 3–8 by their parents and teachers	3; promising research	https://www.cebc4cw.org/program/body-safety-training-workbook/
Parents as Teachers	Primary	Parents with children up to age 5	3; promising research	https://www.cebc4cw.org/program/parents-as-teachers/
Period of Purple Crying	Primary	Parents of infants up to 5 mo of age	3; promising research	https://www.cebc4cw.org/program/period-of-purple-crying/
The Safe Child Program	Primary	Children ages 3–9	3; promising research	https://www.cebc4cw.org/program/the-safe-child-program/
Safe Touches	Primary	Children in kindergarten to third grade	3; promising research	https://www.cebc4cw.org/program/safe-touches/

Program	Level	Target population	Rating	Link
Stewards of Children	Primary	Staff and volunteers of schools or youth serving organizations, parents/caregivers, concerned adults	3; promising research	https://www.cebc4cw.org/program/stewards-of-children/
Strong Communities for Children	Primary	Entire communities	3; promising research	https://www.cebc4cw.org/program/strong-communities-for-children/
Circles of Safety	Primary	Youth-serving organizations	Not able to be rated	https://www.cebc4cw.org/program/circles-of-safety/
Family Hui	Primary	Parents of children up to age 5	Not able to be rated	https://www.cebc4cw.org/program/family-hui/
The Happiest Baby	Primary	New parents, grandparents, teachers and health care professionals	Not able to be rated	https://www.cebc4cw.org/program/the-happiest-baby/
MBF Child/Teen Safety Matters	Primary	Children in grades kindergarten to 12, parents, and school personnel	Not able to be rated	https://www.cebc4cw.org/program/mbf-child-safety-matters/ https://www.cebc4cw.org/program/mbf-teen-safety-matters/
Safe Families for Children	Primary	Parents in crisis and their children up to 18 y of age who need temporary place to live	Not able to be rated	https://www.cebc4cw.org/program/safe-families-for-children-sffc/
The Incredible Years	Secondary	Parents, teachers, and children ages 4–8; versions for high-risk populations	1; well-supported by research evidence	https://www.cebc4cw.org/program/the-incredible-years/
Safe Environment for Every Kid	Secondary	Families with children to age 5 who have risk factors for abuse, such as parental depression or substance abuse	2; supported by research evidence	https://www.cebc4cw.org/program/safe-environment-for-every-kid-seek-model/

(continued on next page)

Table 1
(continued)

Child Welfare Related Program	Type of Prevention	Target Audience	CEBC Rating[a]	Program Information
SafeCare	Secondary	In-home parent training program for at-risk or parents with history of abuse or neglect	2; supported by research evidence	https://www.cebc4cw.org/program/safecare/
C.A.R.E.S (Coordination, Advocacy, Resources, Education and Support)	Secondary	For families at risk for abuse or neglect; parents/caregivers with children up to age 17	3; promising research	https://www.cebc4cw.org/program/c-a-r-e-s-coordination-advocacy-resources-education-and-support/
CICC's Effective Black Parenting Program	Secondary	African-American families at risk for child maltreatment with children up to age 17	3; promising research	https://www.cebc4cw.org/program/effective-black-parenting-program/
Combined Parent-Child Cognitive-Behavioral Therapy	Secondary	For families at risk of physical abuse with children ages 3–17	3; promising research	https://www.cebc4cw.org/program/combined-parent-child-cognitive-behavioral-therapy-cpc-cbt/
Exchange Parent Aide	Secondary	For families at risk with at least one child up to age 12	3; promising research	https://www.cebc4cw.org/program/exchange-parent-aide/
Family Connections	Secondary	For families at risk, parents/caregivers and children up to age 17	3; promising research	https://www.cebc4cw.org/program/family-connections/
Nurturing Parenting Programs for Parents and their School aged Children 5–12 y	Secondary	Families who have been reported to the child welfare system; parents and their school-aged children 5–12 y	3; promising research	https://www.cebc4cw.org/program/nurturing-parenting-program-for-parents-and-their-school-age-children-5-to-12-years/
Step-by-Step Parenting Program	Secondary	Parents with learning differences whose children are at risk of neglect	3; promising research	https://www.cebc4cw.org/program/step-by-step-parenting-program/

CICC's Los Niños Bien Educados	Secondary	Parents of Latino descent who are raising children age 2–12 in the United States	Not able to be rated	https://www.cebc4cw.org/program/los-ninos-bien-educados/
CICC's New Confident Parenting Program	Secondary	Parents of children 2–12 y old, who are experiencing behavior or emotional problems	Not able to be rated	https://www.cebc4cw.org/program/new-confident-parenting-program/
Love and Logic	Secondary	Parents, grandparents, teachers, and other caregivers of children	Not able to be rated	https://www.cebc4cw.org/program/love-and-logic/
Make Parenting A Pleasure 2nd Edition	Secondary	At-risk, highly stressed families with children up to age 8	Not able to be rated	https://www.cebc4cw.org/program/make-parenting-a-pleasure/
Nurturing Parenting Programs for Parents and their Infants, Toddlers, and Preschoolers	Secondary	Families who have been reported to the child welfare system; parents and their infants, toddlers, and preschoolers	Not able to be rated	https://www.cebc4cw.org/program/nurturing-parenting-program-for-parents-and-their-infants-toddlers-and-preschoolers/
Steps Toward Effective, Enjoyable Parenting	Secondary	Home visits and group sessions for first-time, low-income mothers of children up to age 2	Not able to be rated	https://www.cebc4cw.org/program/steps-to-effective-enjoyable-parenting/

[a] This scale is a 1 to 5 rating of the strength of the research evidence supporting a practice or program. A scientific rating of 1 represents a practice with the strongest research evidence and a 5 represents a concerning practice that seems to pose substantial risk to children and families. Some programs do not currently have strong enough research evidence to be rated on the Scientific Rating Scale and are classified as "not able to be rated."

Data from California Evidence-Based Clearinghouse for Child Welfare (CEBC). Available at: http://www.cebc4cw.org. Accessed June 6, 2019.

appropriate caregivers can be addressed with parents. For example, parents of infants can be given information from the National Center on Shaken Baby Syndrome,[31] including coursework their babysitter can complete. Parents of older children and teenagers may benefit from reading a guide produced by the Center for Behavioral Intervention in Beaverton Oregon, Protecting Your Children: Advice from Child Molesters.[32]

- Prevention of CSA is largely school-based and involves the children themselves.[33,34]

Prevention of Abuse Recurrence

Suspicion and identification of child abuse includes recognition of risk factors and physical findings. Many signs of physical abuse may be detected on careful inspection of an undressed child. Health care professionals must perform comprehensive physical examinations of children, including examination of the scalp, skin, oropharynx, and genitalia to identify potential injuries.[35] Comprehensive examinations allow for detection of injuries, such as bruises in unusual locations based on a child's developmental age. It is helpful to recall, "those who don't cruise, rarely bruise."[36]

TEN-4 FACES is a clinical decision tool for bruises that may be helpful to health care professionals.[37] This tool predicts physical abuse (96% sensitivity and 87% specificity) with bruising anywhere on a child less than 4 months old or bruising in a child less than 4 years old on the torso, ears, neck, frenulum, angle of jaw, cheek, or eyelid or subconjunctival hemorrhage. A comprehensive screening instrument for all forms of child abuse is needed and should be a research priority.

Sentinel injuries

The term "sentinel injury" is defined by many child abuse pediatricians as a medically minor injury suspicious for abuse, and therefore, with potential for forensic significance.[38] Minor abusive injuries in precruising infants herald the possibility of more severe future physical abuse.[39,40] Bruising is the most common type of sentinel injury (80%) followed by intraoral injury (11%) and fracture (7%).[37]

Sheets and coworkers[38] reported 27.5% of children determined to have been abused had a previously documented sentinel injury. Health care professionals were aware of a sentinel injury in 42% of abused children. In some cases, providers suspected abuse and reported to the appropriate investigative authorities, yet the child was not protected for a variety of reasons and went on to sustain additional injuries. In other cases, the provider noted the finding, but did not suspect abuse, or the provider stated the injury was consistent with an accidental or self-inflicted mechanism.[38] These data suggest the need for education of health care professionals about significance of sentinel injuries.

Occult and Missed Abuse Injuries

AHT and abusive fractures are missed 30% and 20% of the time, respectively.[39,40] Missed abuse puts children at risk for future, escalating episodes of abuse.[39–41] Radiologic studies, such as skeletal survey and neuroimaging, diagnostic testing, such as hepatic transaminases, and a dilated ophthalmologic examination can identify occult injuries. Identification of occult injuries can increase the rate of abuse recognition.[39–41] Appropriate and timely diagnosis of abuse improves safety planning by investigative workers, such as Department of Social Services and law enforcement. Despite available screening guidelines for occult injuries, there is significant variability in evaluations for child abuse among hospitals and individual health care professionals.[41] Use of protocols for children with sentinel injuries is expected to reduce missed abuse.[42]

Risk of Morbidity and Mortality

Physical abuse may lead to death immediately following the injuries or many years or decades later, related to complications from abuse. At least 1500 children die from child maltreatment in the United States every year.[43] In 2012, Congress passed the Protect Our Kids Act and created the Commission to Eliminate Child Abuse and Neglect Fatalities (CECANF) to address this issue. Berger and colleagues[43] published a perspective article on this in 2015, and in 2016 CECANF published its final report, *Within Our Reach: A National Strategy to Eliminate Child Abuse and Neglect Fatalities.*[44] The following list highlights key recommendations:

- Compared with other age groups, abused infants and toddlers are at high risk for fatality.
- A call to a child protection hotline predicts later abuse or neglect fatalities, regardless of the disposition. Screening out calls may miss children who may be at a high risk.
- Health care and public health agency professionals' involvement is vital to children's safety. Interagency coordination is critical.
- The importance of child protection workers' access to real-time information about families is of great value for the protection of children. Primary care providers often have access to much of this information.
- Accurate data allow a better understanding of what works and what does not.
- The Nurse-Family Partnership program has saved lives.[45]

Reporting and Treating Child Maltreatment

Forty-eight states, the District of Columbia, American Samoa, Guam, the Northern Mariana Islands, Puerto Rico, and the Virgin Islands designate by law all physicians, nurses, and other health care workers who have frequent contact with children as mandated reporters. Approximately 18 states and Puerto Rico require any person, regardless of profession, to report abuse or neglect if suspected.[46] Health care providers must be aware of the laws in their region.

To protect maltreated children, reporting laws in most states restrict a mandated reporter's "privileged communications," the right to maintain confidential communications between professionals and their patients. Although the mandated reporter may choose to remain anonymous in most states, it is helpful to the investigation to know the reporter's identity. The identity of the reporter is not disclosed to the alleged perpetrator in most states. The 2016 factsheet, *Mandatory Reporters of Child Abuse and Neglect*, by the Child Welfare Information Gateway provides the statutes for specific states or territories.[46]

In January 2019 the bipartisan Victims of Child Abuse Reauthorization Act (VOCARA) was signed into law. This law, originally known as the Victims of Child Abuse Act of 1990, initially authorized funding to Children's Advocacy Centers to help victims of child abuse. The 2019 version of this law contains language that further supports the role of health care professionals who provide primary care to children. For many years, mandated reporters have had immunity from legal action if a report was made "in good faith." VOCARA provides the same legal protections to health care professionals who assist with investigations of cases of suspected child maltreatment (eg, a pediatric hospitalist who admits a suspected victim of child abuse and subsequently orders radiographs). This law addresses the trend of pediatricians, and in particular child abuse pediatricians, who are confronted with legal action for their roles in a child's medical evaluation for abuse.[47]

Prevention of Child Sexual Abuse

A multifaceted prevention approach is necessary to address the public health challenge of CSA. Traditionally, tertiary prevention approaches have been used for treatment after an offense occurred, both for survivors of CSA to reduce long-term effects of CSA and its recurrence and for offending individuals. Interventions are needed at primary and secondary prevention levels to treat and support those at risk of sexually offending.[48] Effective primary prevention aimed at potential victims reaches children across all ages beginning with early development of social emotional health. In addition, it tasks adults with developing methods to change social norms and behaviors and to intervene before abuse occurs. Secondary prevention programs target populations at-risk, such as those homeless or under economic stress, children of parents with a mental illness or drug dependency, and LGBTQ+ youth.

Effective prevention efforts require recognition of risk and protective factors at the level of the individual, community, or a society (**Table 2**). Clinical implications of systemic risk factors for the child, parent, family, and community include developing risk assessment strategies and care needs assessments, and to identify those in need of preventive care and what care may be needed.[49]

Expectations for Medical Professionals

Pediatricians have long reported giving inconsistent anticipatory guidance to patients and families about sexual abuse, are uncomfortable discussing sexual issues, were not trained to recognize red flags for sexual abuse, and do not have a consistent approach to cases of suspected abuse.[50] Medical professionals unknowingly see pediatric patients affected by sexual abuse and must be familiar with its definition, including recognition of healthy, concerning, or abusive behaviors, and an understanding of the unique dynamics related to CSA, such as grooming evolution and disclosures.

Prevention before abuse occurs is ideal. Identification of CSA may offer protection from revictimization. Limited CSA screening tools either evaluate behavior and identify symptoms, or identify at-risk youth.

Definition of Child Sexual Abuse

Prevention of CSA requires an understanding of the definition and dynamics of sexual abuse. As defined by the 1999 World Health Organization Consultation on Child Abuse Prevention, "child sexual abuse is the involvement of a child in sexual activity that he or she does not fully comprehend, is unable to give informed consent to, or for which the child is not developmentally prepared and cannot give consent, or that violates the laws or social taboos of society. Child sexual abuse is evidenced by this activity between a child and an adult or another child who by age or development is in a relationship of responsibility, trust, or power, with the activity being intended to gratify or satisfy the needs of the other person. This may include, but is not limited to: the inducement or coercion of a child to engage in any unlawful sexual activity; the exploitative use of a child in prostitution or other unlawful sexual practices; or the exploitative use of children in pornographic performance and materials."[51]

Grooming

Understanding the dynamics of CSA helps to improve health care provider identification of suspected cases and enable intervention before escalation of sexual abuse

Table 2
Risk and protective factors for CSA victimization

	Individual/Interpersonal/Family	Community/Organization	Society
Risk factors	Prior CSA victimization of child and/or siblings, other family members	Poverty	Social climate that tolerates sexual abuse
	Prior or concurrent forms of child abuse in the home	Youth serving organization setting	Insufficient laws and policies
	Parental problems, such as domestic violence, nonconnectedness, nonnuclear family structure, in foster care	"Virtual" settings, cyber-interactions	
	Parental problems, such as domestic violence, nonconnectedness, nonnuclear family structure, in foster care	Lack of institutional support from police and judicial system	
	Poor parent-child relationship, child isolation		
	Female gender		
	Situational factors		
Protective factors and resilience	Presence of caring and supportive adult	Structured, positive school environment	Access to affordable quality health care, including mental health, and social welfare services
	Parental monitoring	Involvement in religious community	Adequate laws and policies
	Social support and connectedness	Involvement in extracurricular activities or hobbies	Research and training programs, public awareness, and education
	Attributes of positive disposition or temperament of child, including strong cognitive ability, internal locus of control, ego control, high self-esteem, spirituality		

Data from Refs.[2,49,61]

behaviors. This includes knowledge of grooming, which builds trust by a perpetrator, who may be a known and trusted caregiver.[52]

Grooming behaviors may include

- Subtle approaches designed to build relationships
- Catering to a child's interests
- Created opportunities to be alone with a child or children
- Special privileges/gifts/favoritism

Disclosure

Children may not disclose an act because of pressure by the perpetrator, concern of consequences, fear of not being believed, lack of opportunity, or a lack of understanding of CSA. A high percentage of sexually abused children hold disclosure until adulthood; therefore, health care professionals can expect to encounter children and adolescents who are withholding disclosure.[53] Implementation of organizational-level protocols ensures quick and supportive responses to disclosure and connects the child to professional services to keep the child safe and facilitate recovery from trauma.

Trafficking

Child victims of labor and sex trafficking are often difficult to identify and have complex medical and mental health needs. National legislation, Stop, Observe, Ask and Respond (SOAR) to Health and Wellness Act, directs the US Department of Health & Human Services to provide health care professionals with training on how to identify and appropriately treat human trafficking victims. There is a need for standardization to ensure accuracy of information, use of trauma-informed and patient-centered care, and consistent messaging. A six-item questionnaire has been shown to be effective in identifying commercial sexual exploitation of children and child sex trafficking victims among a high-risk adolescent population.[54]

Health systems can meet the health care needs of victims by[55–57]

- Providing trafficking training to educate practitioners
- Documenting suspected and confirmed trafficking using International Classification of Diseases-10-US codes
- Establishing an internal response protocol with trauma-informed/patient-centered care
- Implementing an information and referral network for local services offered
- Conspicuously posting the National Human Trafficking Hotline
- Investing in community advocacy, including funding and/or time toward anti-human trafficking initiatives

Prevention of Peer Victimization and Social Media Risks

Peer victimization and child abuse via social media have become areas of grave concern.[58–60] Bullying of children by peers is known to cause mental health, physical, and long-term health consequences, including depression, suicidal ideation, and/or suicide attempts. There is a strong association of cyberbullying with suicide, above and beyond the effects of traditional bullying. Cyberbullying, defined by Kowalski and coworkers,[58] is "the use of electronic communication technologies to bully others."

Social media risks go beyond typical face-to-face bullying, including amplifying and creating a widespread pervasive abusive environment. Tactics can include harassment, humiliation, and other cruel intents. The added risks associated with activated global positioning systems (GPS) satellite services enables perpetrators to find vulnerable children who use GPS applications (eg, Pokémon Go, or dating applications, such as Tinder). However, GPS has many positive uses, including enabling parents to track their children's whereabouts. Likewise, social media can provide important educational and emotional support for children and their parents. Prevention of cyberbullying and the reduction of the risks and harm of social media to children and adolescents requires oversight and vigilance by parents and caregivers.

To identify risks for bullying and cyberbullying, the provider can incorporate some broad questions and discussions, such as asking about experiences with social media, use and types of smart-phone applications, and about observations regarding peers who may be having problems online.[59]

It has been traditionally believed that schools should be responsible for implementing bullying interventions. However, cyberbullying does not just take place in schools and online activities can take place anywhere. The health effects are significant. Hutson[60] recommends that providers use evidence-based, effective programming commonly implemented by schools, such as teaching communication/social skills, empathy training, coping skills, and education on digital citizenship. This is provided through referral for mental health support, or directly by the health care provider. Parents and children should be part of interventions.[60]

SUMMARY

Opportunities to prevent child maltreatment and abuse can be integrated into the pediatric health care visit. Providers should take a broad view of the social, emotional, structural, and family context to identify risks for abuse. Key areas include the public health framework, including support systems that are available to parents. It is important to recognize risk factors for abuse and potential examination findings of physical abuse (especially sentinel injuries) to intervene and prevent further abuse. Sexual abuse prevention is challenging and recognition of signs, including signs of trafficking and peer victimization, requires vigilance. Mandated reporters are protected from liability by federal law as long as they make a report "in good faith." Expansion of this law provides further protection for health care professionals who evaluate and treat suspected child abuse victims.

DISCLOSURE

The authors have nothing to disclose.

REFERENCES

1. Dubowitz H, Feigelman S, Lane W, et al. Pediatric primary care to help prevent child maltreatment: the safe environment for every kid (SEEK) model. Pediatrics 2009;123(3):858–64.
2. Flaherty EG, Stirling J. The pediatrician's role in child maltreatment prevention. Pediatrics 2010;126(4):833.
3. U.S. Preventive Services Task Force. Interventions to Prevent Child Maltreatment: Recommendation Statement. Am Fam Physician 2019;100(2):110–2.
4. U.S. Department of Health & Human Services. Administration for Children & Families, Children's Bureau, Child Welfare Information Gateway. Framework for Prevention of Child Maltreatment. 2017. Available at: https://www.childwelfare.gov/topics/preventing/overview/framework/. Accessed April 25, 2019.
5. Harden BJ, Buhler A, Parra LJ. Maltreatment in infancy: a developmental perspective on prevention and intervention. Trauma Violence Abuse 2016; 17(4):366–86.
6. Flaherty EG, Legano L, Idzerda S. Ongoing pediatric health care for the child who has been maltreated. Pediatrics 2019;143(4):e20190284.
7. Chen M, Chan KL. Effects of parenting programs on child maltreatment prevention: a meta-analysis. Trauma Violence Abuse 2016;17(1):88–104.
8. Pelton LH. The continuing role of maternal factors in child maltreatment and placement. Child Abuse Negl 2015;41:30–9.
9. Lane WG. Prevention of child maltreatment. Pediatr Clin North Am 2014;61(5): 873–88.

10. U.S. Department of Health and Human Services, Administration on Children, Youth and Families. Child maltreatment 2017. Available at: https://www.acf.hhs.gov/sites/default/files/cb/cm2017.pdf. Accessed April 25, 2019.

11. Barr RG, Barr M, Fujiwara T, et al. Do educational materials change knowledge and behaviour about crying and shaken baby syndrome? A randomized controlled trial. CMAJ 2009;180(7):727–33.

12. Barr RG, Trent RB, Cross J. Age-related incidence curve of hospitalized shaken baby syndrome cases: convergent evidence for crying as a trigger to shaking. Child Abuse Negl 2006;30(1):7–16.

13. Goulet C, Frappier JY, Fortin S, et al. Development and evaluation of a shaken baby syndrome prevention program. J Obstet Gynecol Neonatal Nurs 2009; 38(1):7–21.

14. Showers J. "Don't shake the baby": the effectiveness of a prevention program. Child Abuse Negl 1992;16(1):11–8.

15. Altman RL, Canter J, Patrick PA, et al. Parent education by maternity nurses and prevention of abusive head trauma. Pediatrics 2011;128(5):e1164–72.

16. Dias MS, Rottmund CM, Cappos KM, et al. Association of a postnatal parent education program for abusive head trauma with subsequent pediatric abusive head trauma hospitalization rates. JAMA Pediatr 2017;171(3):223–9.

17. Lyons SJ, Henly JR, Schuerman JR. Informal support in maltreating families: its effect on parenting practices. Child Youth Serv Rev 2005;27:21–38.

18. Colemen PK, Karraker KH. Self-efficacy and parenting quality: findings and future applications. Developmental Rev 1998;18:47–85.

19. Runyan DK, Hunter WM, Socolar RR, et al. Children who prosper in unfavorable environments: the relationship to social capital. Pediatrics 1998;101(1 Pt 1):12–8.

20. Dubowitz H. The safe environment for every kid model: promotion of children's health, development, and safety, and prevention of child neglect. Pediatr Ann 2014;43(11):e271–7.

21. Dubowitz H, Lane WG, Semiatin JN, et al. The safe environment for every kid model: impact on pediatric primary care professionals. Pediatrics 2011;127(4): e962–70.

22. California Department of Social Services, Office of Child Abuse Prevention. The California evidence-based clearinghouse for child welfare. 2019. Available at: https://www.cebc4cw.org/. Accessed June 6, 2019.

23. Breiner H, Ford M, Gadsden VL, editors. Parenting matters: supporting parents of children ages 0-8. Washington, DC: National Academy of Sciences; 2016.

24. Olds DL. Preventing child maltreatment and crime with prenatal and infancy support of parents: the nurse-family partnership. J Scand Stud Criminol Crime Prev 2008;9(S1):2–24.

25. Vlahovicova K, Melendez-Torres GJ, Leijten P, et al. Parenting programs for the prevention of child physical abuse recurrence: a systematic review and meta-analysis. Clin Child Fam Psychol Rev 2017;20(3):351–65.

26. Nurse-Family Partnership. Nurse-Family Partnership Web site. 2019. Available at: https://www.nursefamilypartnership.org/first-time-moms/. Accessed June 20, 2019.

27. American Academy of Pediatrics. Connected Kids: Safe, Strong, Secure. 2019. Available at: https://www.aap.org/en-us/advocacy-and-policy/aap-health-initiatives/Pages/Connected-Kids.aspx. Accessed June 17, 2019.

28. American Academy of Pediatrics. Practicing Safety Program. 2019. Available at: https://www.aap.org/en-us/advocacy-and-policy/aap-health-initiatives/practicing-safety/Pages/Phase-I.aspx. Accessed June 6, 2019.

29. Child Abuse Medical Provider Program. Staying positive while parenting. CHAMP Program Web site. 2019. Available at: http://champprogram.com/pdf/Staying-Positive-While-Parenting-pamphlet.pdf. Accessed June 19, 2019.

30. Centers for Disease Control and Prevention. Technical packages for violence prevention: using evidence-based strategies in your violence prevention efforts. 2019. Available at: https://www.cdc.gov/violenceprevention/pub/technical-packages.html. Accessed June 22, 2019.

31. National Center on Shaken Baby Syndrome. Available courses. 2019. Available at: https://training.dontshake.org/courses. Accessed June 18, 2019.

32. The Center for Behavioral Intervention in Beaverton, Oregon. Protecting your children: advice from child molesters. Vermont Official State Website: Agency of Human Services Department for Children and Families Web site. 2019. Available at: https://dcf.vermont.gov/sites/dcf/files/Prevention/docs/Protecting-Children.pdf. Accessed June 15, 2019.

33. Black DA, Heyman RE, Smith Slep AM. Risk factors for child sexual abuse. Aggress Violent Behav 2001;6(2):203–29.

34. Davis MK, Gidycz CA. Child sexual abuse prevention programs: a meta-analysis. J Clin Child Psychol 2000;29(2):257–65.

35. Christian CW. The evaluation of suspected child physical abuse. Pediatrics 2015; 135(5):e1337–54.

36. Sugar NF, Taylor JA, Feldman KW. Bruises in infants and toddlers: those who don't cruise rarely bruise. Puget Sound Pediatric Research Network. Arch Pediatr Adolesc Med 1999;153(4):399–403.

37. Clyde Pierce M, Kaczor K, Aldridge A, et al. Bruising characteristics discriminating physical child abuse from accidental trauma. Pediatrics 2010;125(1): 67–74.

38. Sheets LK, Leach ME, Koszewski IJ, et al. Sentinel injuries in infants evaluated for child physical abuse. Pediatrics 2013;131(4):701–7.

39. Jenny C, Hymel KP, Ritzen A, et al. Analysis of missed cases of abusive head trauma. JAMA 1999;281(7):621–6.

40. Ravichandiran N, Schuh S, Bejuk M, et al. Delayed identification of pediatric abuse-related fractures. Pediatrics 2010;125(1):60–6.

41. Wood JN, Feudtner C, Medina SP, et al. Variation in occult injury screening for children with suspected abuse in selected US children's hospitals. Pediatrics 2012;130(5):853–60.

42. Lindberg DM, Juarez-Colunga E, Wood JN, et al. Testing for abuse in children with sentinel injuries. Pediatrics 2015;136(5):831–8.

43. Berger RP, Sanders D, Rubin D. Commission to Eliminate Abuse and Neglect Fatalities. Pediatricians' role in preventing child maltreatment fatalities: a call to action. Pediatrics 2015;136(5):825–7.

44. U.S. Department of Health & Human Services. Administration for children & families, children's bureau, commission to eliminate child abuse and neglect fatalities. Within our reach: a national strategy to eliminate child abuse and neglect fatalities. Washington, DC: Government Printing Office; 2016. Available at: http://www.acf.hhs.gov/programs/cb/resource/cecanf-final-report, 2016. Accessed on March 19, 2020.

45. Child Welfare League of America. Commission releases final report on child fatalities. 2016. Available at: https://www.cwla.org/commission-releases-final-report-on-child-fatalities/. Accessed June 20, 2019.

46. U.S. Department of Health & Human Services. Administration for Children & Families, Children's Bureau, Child Welfare Information Gateway. Mandatory reporters

of child abuse and neglect. 2017. Available at: https://www.childwelfare.gov/pubpdfs/manda.pdf. Accessed April 25, 2019.

47. Library of the Congress. Victims of Child Abuse Act Reauthorization Act of 2018. 2018. Available at: https://www.congress.gov/bill/115th-congress/senate-bill/2961/all-info. Accessed July 24, 2019.

48. Knack N, Winder B, Murphy L, et al. Primary and secondary prevention of child sexual abuse. Int Rev Psychiatry 2019;31(2):181–94.

49. Assink M, van der Put CE, Meeuwsen MWCM, et al. Risk factors for child sexual abuse victimization: a meta-analytic review. Psychol Bull 2019;145(5):459–89.

50. Leder MR, Emans J, Hafler JP, et al. Addressing sexual abuse in the primary care setting. Pediatrics 1999;104:270–5.

51. World Health Organization. Violence and Injury Prevention Team & Global Forum for Health Research, Consultation on Child Abuse Prevention. Report of the Consultation on Child Abuse Prevention; 1999. Available at: https://apps.who.int/iris/handle/10665/65900. Accessed on March 19, 2020.

52. World Health Organization. Chapter 7, Child Sexual Abuse in Guidelines for medico-legal care of victims of sexual violence. 2003. Gender and Women's Health, Family and Community Health Injuries and Violence Prevention, Noncommunicable Diseases and Mental Health, Geneva, Switzerland.

53. Townsend C. Child sexual abuse disclosure: what practitioners need to know. 2016. Available at: https://www.d2l.org/wp-content/uploads/2016/10/ChildSexualAbuseDisclosurePaper_20160217_v.1.pdf. Accessed June 6, 2019.

54. Greenbaum J, Dodd M, McCracken C. A short screening tool to identify victims of child sex trafficking in the health care setting. Pediatr Emerg Care 2018;34(1):33–7.

55. Greenbaum J, Stoklosa H. The healthcare response to human trafficking: a need for globally harmonized ICD codes. PLoS Med 2019;16(5).

56. Greenbaum J, Crawford-Jakubiak JE. Committee on Child Abuse and Neglect. Child sex trafficking and commercial sexual exploitation: health care needs of victims. Pediatrics 2015;135(3):566–74.

57. Polaris. National Human Trafficking Hotline. 2019. Available at: https://humantrafficking.org/. Accessed June 2, 2019.

58. Kowalski RM, Giumetti GW, Schroeder AN, et al. Bullying in the digital age: a critical review and meta-analysis of cyberbullying research among youth. Psychol Bull 2014;140(4):1073–137.

59. Englander E, Donnerstein E, Kowalski R, et al. Defining cyberbullying. Pediatrics 2017;140(Suppl 2):S148–51.

60. Hutson E. Cyberbullying in adolescence: a concept analysis. ANS Adv Nurs Sci 2016;39(1):60–70.

61. McKillop N. Understanding the nature and dimensions of child sexual abuse to inform its prevention. In: Bryce I, Robinson Y, Petherick W, editors. Child abuse and neglect: forensic issues in evidence, impact and management. Cambridge (MA): Elsevier; 2019. p. 241–59.

Behavioral Approaches to Assessment and Early Intervention for Severe Problem Behavior in Intellectual and Developmental Disabilities

Patricia F. Kurtz, PhD[a,b], Mauro Leoni, PhD[c,d],
Louis P. Hagopian, PhD, BCBA-D[a,b],*

KEYWORDS

- Severe problem behavior • Intellectual disability • Applied behavior analysis
- Behavioral assessment and treatment • Early intervention

KEY POINTS

- Problem behavior occurs in 50% of children with intellectual and developmental disabilities; in 10% of cases, problem behavior is considered severe.
- Risk factors for problem behavior include presence of more severe intellectual disability, a diagnosis of autism, sensory impairments, and deficits in communication.
- Functional analysis and function-based treatments based on the principles of applied behavior analysis are considered best practices.
- Pediatricians play a crucial role in early identification of problem behavior, referral to early intervention services, and parent education.

PHENOMENOLOGY OF PROBLEM BEHAVIOR
Description and Prevalence

Children with intellectual and developmental disabilities (IDDs) are at increased risk for problem behavior.[1] A subset of these individuals develop severe problem behavior, which can pose serious and immediate risk for injury, loss of function, disfigurement, and even death.[2] Self-injurious behavior (SIB) includes behaviors such as head-

[a] Neurobehavioral Unit, Kennedy Krieger Institute, 707 North Broadway, Baltimore, MD 21205, USA; [b] Department of Psychiatry and Behavioral Sciences, Johns Hopkins University School of Medicine, Baltimore, MD, USA; [c] Department of Disabilities, Fondazione Istituto Ospedaliero di Sospiro Onlus, Piazza Libertà, 2, Sospiro (CR) 26048, Italy; [d] Freud University of Milan, Italy
* Corresponding author. Neurobehavioral Unit, Kennedy Krieger Institute, 707 North Broadway, Baltimore, MD 21205.
E-mail address: hagopian@kennedykrieger.org

Pediatr Clin N Am 67 (2020) 499–511
https://doi.org/10.1016/j.pcl.2020.02.005
0031-3955/20/© 2020 Elsevier Inc. All rights reserved.

banging, head hitting, self-biting, and self-scratching. These can cause localized swelling, bruising, and bleeding; loss of tissue from tongue, lips, ears, and nose; blindness from retinal detachment; and permanent disfigurement.[3] Aggressive and disruptive behaviors can reach comparable levels of severity and result in severe injuries to family members and staff.[4] Pica (the ingestion of nonedible items) and elopement (leaving a supervised area without caregiver knowledge) can result in injury or death.[5]

Estimates vary widely, but approximately 50% of individuals with IDD experience some form of problem behavior, with a smaller proportion (5%–10%) exhibiting very severe problem behavior with extreme consequences for families and caregivers.[6–8] These problems appear to be more common among individuals with IDD who also have autism spectrum disorder (ASD).[4,9] Other known risk factors for problem behavior include greater deficits in intellectual functioning and communication, and the presence of sensory impairments.[1,10] Recently identified risk markers include repetitive and restricted behavior and interests, overactivity/impulsivity,[11,12] and prenatal factors (level of maternal education, maternal smoking, and electronic fetal monitoring during labor) associated with SIB in children with ASD.[13,14]

In this population, problem behavior is a heterogeneous phenomenon. Onset of problem behavior may occur in early childhood or adolescence, or adulthood in some cases. Individuals may present with one type of problem behavior or may engage in multiple forms. These behaviors can occur from dozens to hundreds of times daily or episodically. Problem behaviors sometimes co-occur with irritability or in the context of an outburst where there also are expressions of anger, frustration, and other negative emotional states.[15] Because these behaviors can vary greatly in their complexity and intensity, so does their impact on children and families. When problem behaviors occur regularly, and with high intensity, they might produce injuries to self or others, restrict participation in activities appropriate for the individual's developmental level, and necessitate a higher level of care (constant supervision, multiple people required to manage problem behavior when an episode occurs, and so forth) and increased emergency room visits.[16] As a result of these many challenges, it is more likely that medication is overprescribed for this population with poor efficacy and high risk of negative side effects.[17,18] When these behaviors are severe and persistent, they can lead to mistreatment, including inappropriate restraint and seclusion,[19] expulsion from school, placement in restrictive settings, and occurrence of physical and emotional trauma to family members.[20–22] Family members often report feeling isolated, and financial resources are strained as a result of additional expenses.

Establishment of Problem Behavior

Problem behavior in this population is thought to be the product of the interaction between deficits stemming from IDD and experiences that reinforce and strengthen these behaviors.[23,24] Deficits in communication and adaptive skills and limited ability to regulate emotions may increase the frequency and intensity of frustrative experiences, setting the stage for episodes of irritability and problem behavior. Because problem behavior often is dangerous or socially unacceptable, caregivers understandably work to calm children via redirection, consolation, or interruption.[25] For example, if a child engages in SIB when presented with instructional demands, the caregiver may give the child a break in an attempt to calm the child and avoid injury or disruption of the environment. Although well-intended, these reactions sometimes may reinforce the problem through basic learning processes and thus increase its future occurrence. Caregivers sometimes also actively work to avoid situations that might cause distress by altering their routines—but if this process of accommodation continues and expands to other situations, then altered routines to avoid challenging situations may become highly disruptive to the point they are unsustainable.[26] Thus, although efforts to make problem behavior cease or to avoid situations that occasion it may provide some immediate relief to the caregiver, such interactions can lead to the establishment and maintenance of maladaptive caregiver-child interaction patterns.[25,27–29] These interaction patterns can impair functioning further as the avoidance of potentially challenging situations expands over time and across settings and becomes a source of chronic stress for parents.

BEHAVIORAL ASSESSMENT AND TREATMENT OF PROBLEM BEHAVIOR

For any given case, the historical events that led to establishment of problem behavior may be difficult if not impossible to identify. Functional behavioral assessment is acknowledged to be the best approach to precisely identify events in the environment that presently occasion problem behavior (antecedents) and the reinforcers that strengthen and maintain those behaviors (consequences). Once identified, knowledge of these controlling events can inform the development of individualized behavioral interventions that are directly tied to the variables that maintain the behavior. Such knowledge also can contribute to identifying what other elements of the clinical presentation should be targeted with pharmacologic interventions, including emotion dysregulation, irritability, hyperactivity, and so forth.[30,31]

Applied Behavior Analysis

Applied behavior analysis (ABA) is a discipline that utilizes principles of learning and behavioral science for the purpose of addressing problems of social significance.[32] ABA-based treatment for addressing the needs of persons with IDD has 2 broad domains of application: (1) educational treatment delivered in the context of a comprehensive intervention and (2) problem-focused treatment, aimed at addressing specific problems. Comprehensive ABA intervention is broad in its scope, aimed at establishing educational and adaptive skills to have an impact on global measures of functioning when applied over an extended period (30+ service hours per week, over a span of years is not uncommon). When implemented early, comprehensive treatment often is referred to using the term, *early intensive behavioral intervention*.[33–35] Problem-focused ABA interventions are more relevant to the current discussion on problem behavior, because these are aimed at addressing more specific problems—most typically, problem behavior, such as SIB, aggression toward others, pica, disruptive behavior, and elopement. Problem-focused interventions are more targeted and, therefore, more time-limited. The goal of these interventions is reducing problem behavior while also establishing and strengthening adaptive behaviors. Some individuals may require both types of ABA treatment. Despite their differences, both comprehensive and problem-focused ABA interventions are based on the same empirically validated learning principles, which involve the objective measurement of behavior using direct observation of behavior, carefully controlling environmental variables for the purpose of pinpointing specific determinants of the severe problem behavior to inform treatment development, and isolating operative components of behavioral interventions.

Empirical Support for Applied Behavior Analysis

Both comprehensive and problem-focused ABA treatments have a strong base of empirical support. Group designs (including randomized controlled trials) have been used to evaluate comprehensive ABA treatment,[34] and single-case experimental designs have been extensively used to document problem-focused ABA interventions (assessment and treatment of problem behavior). Several meta-analyses have examined ABA problem-focused interventions for decreasing rates of various types of problem behavior (eg, see Hayaert and colleagues[36] and Harvey and colleagues[37]). Structured evaluative reviews also have demonstrated that ABA-based approaches are efficacious for aggression,[38] SIB,[39] elopement,[40] and, more broadly, severe problem behavior.[41,42] Problem-focused ABA treatment of problem behavior also has been supported by the Autism Evidence-Based Practice Review Group[43] and the National Standards Project.[44]

Functional Behavioral Assessment

As applied to the assessment and treatment of problem behavior, problem-focused ABA relies heavily on functional behavior assessment. Functional behavior assessment involves a range of techniques aimed at identifying the variables that occasion and maintain problem behavior. Rating scales, interviews, and observations of problem behavior in uncontrolled naturalistic settings and controlled formal assessments can be performed. Generally, less-intensive assessment procedures should be used initially (ie, interviews and rating scales), reserving more time and resource-intensive assessments if less-intensive procedures fail to produce clear assessment findings or lead to the development of an effective intervention. Research on methods that rely on the reporting of others shows they have limited validity relative to methods involving direct observation of behavior. A formal controlled functional analysis, in which conditions are systematically manipulated, is the most valid and scientifically rigorous method of assessment because it directly examines how problem behavior changes as environmental antecedents and consequences are systematically altered.[45] For example, if a child's problem behavior is hypothesized to be maintained by attention from a caregiver, the test condition would involve arranging a situation in which the caregiver provides a form of attention (e.g., telling child to stop, consoling him/her) whenever the problem behavior occurs. In the control condition in this case, the caregiver interacts with the child, without providing attention for problem behavior.

Classification of problem behavior is based on its function, which includes 2 broad classes, both of which include subclasses: (1) socially maintained (occasioned and reinforced through the interactions of others) and (2) automatically maintained (occurs independent of social contingencies). SIB is socially maintained in two-thirds to three-fourths of cases and automatically maintained in one-fourth of cases.[46–48] Aggression most often is socially maintained, whereas pica most often is automatically maintained.[49] Within the broad class of socially maintained problem behavior, the subclasses include problem behavior maintained by (1) attention from adults or peers, (2) escape from or avoiding unpleasant circumstances (eg, demands placed on them by a parent or teacher), and (3) acquiring or gaining access to preferred items, activities, and so forth. In contrast, automatically maintained problem behavior persists independent of interactions with others and presumably via some unknown biological process. That is, the act of engaging in the problem behavior directly produces consequences independent of social interaction that are presumed to be reinforcing in some way.

Function-Based Treatment

Function-based treatment represents best practices in ABA.[46] With knowledge of the controlling variables of problem behavior, precisely targeted interventions can be devised. Broadly speaking, this approach involves 2 primary components designed to (1) strengthen appropriate alternative behaviors (using reinforcement) concurrently with (2) the withholding of reinforcement that maintains the targeted problem behavior (operant extinction). One of the most commonly researched treatments of problem behavior maintained by social consequences is referred to as *functional communication training* (FCT). FCT involves training a child to emit an appropriate communicative response to access reinforcement in lieu of problem behavior. Described in more than 200 studies, FCT is an empirically supported treatment[50] that also has been shown to be highly effective using meta-analysis[51] and in 3 consecutive-controlled case series studies.[52–54] Noncontingent reinforcement (NCR) is another widely researched function-based treatment that has been demonstrated to be empirically supported treatment using the APA criteria[55] and via meta-analysis.[56] NCR involves the response-independent delivery of reinforcers responsible for maintaining problem behavior at fixed or variable times during treatment, thus attenuating motivation for problem behavior. A range of other ABA problem-focused interventions have been shown to be efficacious (see Hagopian and colleagues[49] for a review).

EARLY INTERVENTION AND PREVENTION

The benefits of early intervention are well documented for children with ASD[57,58] and children with IDD.[59–61] For example, outcome studies on intensive programs for children with ASD that focus on skill acquisition and reduction of behavioral excesses have reported significant improvements, including gains on estimates of intellectual functioning, success in regular education classrooms, and functioning similarly to non-ASD samples.[34,57,58] Similarly, elimination or prevention of problem behavior in young children with IDD permits access to early intervention and preschool programs from which they otherwise might be excluded because these programs are not equipped to deal with severe problem behavior. Such programs have components (teaching cooperation, early language skills, and so forth) that would be particularly beneficial to young, at-risk children. Thus, early intervention for problem behavior is highly cost-effective, relative to costs of intensive treatment, and can produce measurable improvement in long-term outcomes for children with IDD.

As discussed previously, research findings from the field of ABA have shown that patterns of caregiver responding and child communication deficits contribute greatly to the maintenance of severe problem behavior exhibited by individuals with IDD.[48] These findings have been replicated with young children who exhibit SIB and other problem behaviors.[62,63] Outcomes of functional analyses conducted with children as young as 1 year to 6 years indicated that in most cases, problem behavior is maintained by social consequences—consistent with research on older children and adults.[48,64] Treatment using FCT and other function-based interventions (eg, NCR) produced notable reductions in problem behavior and increases in communication and other appropriate behaviors. In addition to the impressive clinical outcome, parents found the behavioral assessment and treatment procedures very acceptable.[65] Thus, best practice procedures, when applied at an early age, can effectively treat severe problem behavior.

In contrast to the extensive research literature on treatment of severe problem behavior, preventing the development of problem behavior has received little attention. Initial studies have applied FCT as a preventive approach with children at risk for development of problem behavior, with promising results. Young children taught communication phrases that were substitutable for common social functions of problem behavior (ie, to obtain adult attention or preferred activities or to escape task demands) showed decreases in minor problem behavior; frequency and severity of problem behavior increased in control group children, demonstrating a preventive effect for FCT.

Recent studies have examined prevention of problem behavior using single-case experimental designs (rather than group designs) because this approach permits precision in within-subject measurement, replication, and control, which has great utility in the initial stages of experimental evaluation of prevention approaches.[66] Sensitivity tests based on functional analysis methods have been developed to screen for the emergence of problem behavior in single cases. Communication training is conducted in the specific contexts where problem behavior is likely to occur, and then a prevention effect of FCT is demonstrated. A laboratory model to study the prevention of development of problem behavior also has been piloted,[67] which integrates basic and applied behavioral research. In sum, these studies suggest that FCT may be a feasible approach to preventing the development of more severe forms of problem behavior.

PEDIATRIC CARE: SURVEILLANCE, PREVENTION, AND EARLY INTERVENTION
Surveillance

In light of the increased risks for children with IDD to display severe problem behavior, ongoing surveillance on the part of pediatricians for the early emergence of this problem is necessary. The presence of genetic conditions that may be associated with problem behavior, the diagnosis of ASD, intellectual and sensory impairments, and deficits in adaptive skills are known risk factors for problem behavior and, therefore, must be assessed to determine the relative risk. Many recommendations on pediatric management of ASD[68-70] also are applicable to the broader population of children with IDD. Awareness of the family's social supports, resources, and the caregivers' capacity to physically manage problem behavior can inform efforts to seek supports available through insurance or social service organizations. Evaluation of caregiver stress and psychiatric issues also is necessary to guide caregivers to access services necessary to address their needs (**Box 1**).

As discussed previously, problem behavior in IDD stems from the interaction of deficits associated with IDD and the environment. Problem behavior can be difficult to tolerate because it is potentially harmful to the child or others. Consequently, there often is a sense of urgency on the part of caregivers to interrupt problem behavior or even prevent it from occurring. Although sometimes necessary and even helpful, attempts to calm, console, and appease the child also can reinforce and, therefore, maintain the behavior in the long term. Caregivers inadvertently reinforcing problem behavior from time to time may not result in long-term problems, but persistent maladaptive patterns of interaction can be established through reinforcement processes that can increase the occurrence and severity of problem behavior over time. Therefore, the pediatrician has a critical role in educating caregivers about the potential risks related to the emergence of problem behavior to prevent these patterns of interaction from being established and to initiate early intervention efforts rapidly once it appears they are emerging. Surveillance by routinely inquiring about problem behavior at regular visits is essential to identifying emerging problem behavior and caregiver-child interaction patterns that may inadvertently strengthen problem behavior. Caregiver report of problem behavior may be the primary source of information, because some children may be inhibited in the examination room. Children's behavior, however, and a caregiver's reactions to problem behavior in the waiting area and in response to physical examination can be informative. As has been reported in other pediatric populations, including children dealing with chronic medical problems, caregiver responses that are overly indulgent or overly harsh are associated with negative outcomes.

Box 1
Prevention and early intervention for problem behavior

Primary prevention
  Referral for early intervention services for IDDs
    Departments of health and education
  Assessment
    Child's functioning
    Caregiver capacity and resources
  Education of caregivers
    Education of caregivers on increased risk of problem behavior
    Education of caregivers on resources
  Ongoing surveillance for emergence of problem behavior
    Injuries
    Caregiver report
    Observations during clinic visits

Early intervention
  Assessment of problem behavior and caregiver capacity
    Risks of problem behavior
    Caregiver capacity and skills
  Education of caregivers on caregiver-child interaction patterns
  Referral to specialists

Secondary intervention
  Referral to and collaboration with behavior specialists
  Relevant factors to consider related to initiating medication management
    Consider response to behavioral intervention
    Consider risks of problem behavior
    Consider comorbid medical and psychiatric conditions
    Consider level of experience and knowledge
    Consider referral to another physician with specialized expertise
  If medication management is initiated
    Monitor outcomes using objective measures
    Monitor for potential adverse effects
    Monitor regularly, adjusting dosage or medicine based on response

---

Likewise, it also is important to identify what efforts caregivers undertake to avoid situations that occasion problem behavior. Accommodation involves efforts aimed at avoiding situations that could lead to problem behavior, including engaging in routines or activities that are disruptive to family functioning and appeasing a child when it appears problem behavior begins to occur. Although not all accommodations are unreasonable, some can be highly disruptive to functioning to the point they are not sustainable and maintain maladaptive interaction patterns where the child is in charge. Therefore, the level of risk should be based on consideration of injuries incurred, close calls, and the potential for injury based on consideration of how often the behavior occurs, its likely sequelae, and the level of effort necessary to prevent its occurrence.

Early Intervention

Referring caregivers to locally available early intervention services for children with IDD is essential, because these can provide families access to myriad services to promote development and positive caregiver-child interactions. Evidence supporting the efficacy of early intervention for children with ASD is robust. When the presence of problem behavior is evident, assessment of physical risks of problem behavior is important for determining what level of intervention is indicated. Any observation of injuries to a child or caregiver should be discussed. As discussed previously, problem behavior can include aggression, property destruction, SIB, elopement, pica, and other behaviors that pose risk to self and others. Within these different types, there is tremendous variation in both the form of the behavior and risks it may pose. Risk can be determined by the presence of injuries, the nature of the behavior itself, and the inherent risks it poses. Aggression can produce serious injury, anxiety, and post-traumatic stress to caregivers[38]; SIB can result in infection, loss of tissue, permanent disfigurement, and loss of function[39]; pica can necessitate surgery and result in poisoning, asphyxiation, and even death[71]; and elopement can result in injury or death.[5] Caregiver reports of close calls where severe injury was narrowly avoided by caregiver vigilance can indicate level of risk. Likewise, risk also can be ascertained based on a review of what efforts currently are in place to supervise the child and to prevent injury: the more intensive the efforts needed, the greater the risk because such efforts are difficult to sustain over long periods of time (see **Box 1**).

Secondary Intervention

Once problem behavior is determined to be present and warranting intervention, a variety of options often exist. Some school systems provide intensive behavioral services, and some states mandate funding for services for children diagnosed with ASD. Because many states have recognized that ABA is the most empirically supported approach for problem behavior, licensure and funding for behavior analysts have increased the availability of services. If resources available through educational and public early intervention services are insufficient to meet the needs, referral for specialized behavioral services or the use of medication should be considered.[72] Ideally, medication would be applied after a functional behavioral assessment has been conducted to identify environmental antecedents and child-caregiver interactions that may be reinforcing the problem behavior. Aripiprazole and risperidone have Food and Drug Administration approval for treatment of irritability in ASD and have been deemed appropriate to use if problem behavior poses risks to safety or could lead to more restrictive placement or if other interventions have been attempted and failed to produce sufficient improvement. Other medications have limited support for ASD[72] and SIB.[73–77] Pediatricians must determine whether they possess sufficient experience and knowledge to initiate medication management or if referral to another medical professional is appropriate (see **Box 1**).

Although the combined use of medication and basic behavioral intervention requires further study and is not routinely practiced, this approach has been advocated by many. The general premise is that medication and behavioral interventions can work synergistically. Medications may decrease emotional reactivity, irritability, impulsivity, and other sources of dysregulation, whereas behavioral interventions target adaptive skills and alter maladaptive patterns of interactions (see Hagopian and colleagues[30]). In addition, improved regulation produced by medication may increase a child's ability to benefit from behavioral interventions. Finally, if behavioral and pharmacologic interventions are combined, behavioral data being collected to evaluate the behavioral intervention could be used to help evaluate the effects of medications. Whether medication is applied alone or concurrently with behavioral interventions, measuring outcomes in a systematic manner (eg, the Aberrant Behavior Checklist) helps assess outcomes and adverse effects.

DISCLOSURE

The authors have nothing to disclose.

REFERENCES

1. McClintock K, Hall S, Oliver C. Risk markers associated with challenging behaviours in people with intellectual disabilities: A meta-analytic study. J Intellect Disabil Res 2003;47(6):405–16.
2. Hyman SL, Fisher W, Mercugliano M, et al. Children with self-injurious behavior. Pediatrics 1990;85(3):437.
3. Kuhn DE, Hagopian L, Terlonge C. Treatment of life-threatening self-injurious behavior secondary to hereditary sensory and autonomic neuropathy type II: A controlled case study. J Child Neurol 2008;23(4):381–8.
4. Farmer CA, Aman MG. Aggressive behavior in a sample of children with autism spectrum disorders. Res Autism Spectr Disord 2011;5(1):317–23.
5. Anderson C, Law JK, Daniels A, et al. Occurrence and family impact of elopement in children with autism spectrum disorders. Pediatrics 2012;130(5):870–7.
6. Dekker MC, Koot HM, Ende JVD, et al. Emotional and behavioral problems in children and adolescents with and without intellectual disability. J Child Psychol Psychiatry 2002;43(8):1087–98.
7. Emerson E, Kiernan C, Alborz A, et al. The prevalence of challenging behaviors: a total population study. Res Dev Disabil 2001;22(1):77–93.
8. Sturmey P, Seiverling L, Ward-Horner J. 5 - Assessment of challenging behaviors in people with autism spectrum disorders. In: Matson JL, editor. Clinical assessment and intervention for autism spectrum disorders. San Diego (CA): Academic Press; 2008. p. 131–63.
9. Soke G, Rosenberg S, Hamman R, et al. Brief report: Prevalence of self-injurious behaviors among children with autism spectrum disorder—A population-based study. J Autism Dev Disord 2016;46(11):3607–14.
10. Baghdadli A, Pascal C, Grisi S, et al. Risk factors for self-injurious behaviours among 222 young children with autistic disorders. J Intellect Disabil Res 2003; 47(8):622–7.
11. Davies L, Oliver C. Self-injury, aggression and destruction in children with severe intellectual disability: Incidence, persistence and novel, predictive behavioural risk markers. Res Dev Disabil 2016;49:291–301.
12. Petty JL, Bacarese-Hamilton M, Davies LE, et al. Correlates of self-injurious, aggressive and destructive behaviour in children under five who are at risk of developmental delay. Res Dev Disabil 2014;35(1):36–45.
13. Soke GN, Rosenberg SA, Hamman RF, et al. Factors associated with self-injurious behaviors in children with autism spectrum disorder: Findings from two large national samples. J Autism Dev Disord 2017;47(2):285–96.
14. Soke GN, Rosenberg SA, Hamman RF, et al. Prenatal, perinatal, and neonatal factors associated with self-injurious behaviors in children with autism spectrum disorder. Res Autism Spectr Disord 2019;61:1–9.
15. McGuire K, Fung LK, Hagopian L, et al. Irritability and problem behavior in autism spectrum disorder: a practice pathway for pediatric primary care. Pediatrics 2016;137(Supplement 2):S136.
16. Kalb LG, Vasa RA, Ballard ED, et al. Epidemiology of injury-related emergency department visits in the US among youth with autism spectrum disorder. J Autism Dev Disord 2016;46(8):2756–63.
17. Emerson E, Robertson J, Gregory N, et al. Treatment and management of challenging behaviours in residential settings. J Appl Res Intellect Disabil 2000; 13(4):197–215.

18. Sturmey P, Lott JD, Laud R, et al. Correlates of restraint use in an institutional population: a replication. J Intellect Disabil Res 2005;49(7):501–6.
19. Butler J. How safe is the schoolhouse?: an analysis of state seclusion and restraint laws and policies. Autism National Committee; 2012.
20. Hauser-Cram P, Warfield ME, Shonkoff JP, et al. A Longitudinal study of child development and parent well-being. Monogr Soc Res Child Dev 2001;66(3):i–viii, 1–114; [discussion: 115–26].
21. McIntyre LL, Blacher J, Baker BL. Behaviour/mental health problems in young adults with intellectual disability: The impact on families. J Intellect Disabil Res 2002;46(3):239–49.
22. Neece CL, Green SA, Baker BL. Parenting stress and child behavior problems: a transactional relationship across time. Am J Intellect Dev Disabil 2012;117(1): 48–66.
23. Furniss F, Biswas A. Recent research on aetiology, development and phenomenology of self-injurious behaviour in people with intellectual disabilities: a systematic review and implications for treatment. J Intellect Disabil Res 2012;56(5): 453–75.
24. Oliver C, Adams D, Allen D, et al. Causal models of clinically significant behaviors in Angelman, Cornelia de Lange, Prader-Willi and Smith Magenis syndromes. Int Rev Res Dev Disabil 2013;44:167–211.
25. Stocco CS, Thompson RH. Contingency analysis of caregiver behavior: Implications for parent training and future directions. J Appl Behav Anal 2015;48(2): 417–35.
26. Storch EA, Zavrou S, Collier AB, et al. Preliminary study of family accommodation in youth with autism spectrum disorders and anxiety: Incidence, clinical correlates, and behavioral treatment response. J Anxiety Disord 2015;34:94–9.
27. Addison L, Lerman DC. Descriptive analysis of teachers'responses to problem behavior following training. J Appl Behav Anal 2009;42(2):485–90.
28. Carr EG, Taylor JC, Robinson S. The effects of severe behavior problems in children on the teaching behavior of adults. J Appl Behav Anal 1991;24(3):523–35.
29. Sloman KN, Vollmer TR, Cotnoir NM, et al. Descriptive analyses of caregiver reprimands. J Appl Behav Anal 2005;38(3):373–83.
30. Hagopian L, Caruso-Anderson M. Integrating behavioral and pharmacological interventions for severe problem behavior displayed by children with neurogenetic and developmental disorders. Neurogenetic Syndromes: Behavioral Issues and Their Treatment 2010:217–39.
31. Wachtel LE, Hagopian LP. Psychopharmacology and applied behavioral analysis: tandem treatment of severe problem behaviors in intellectual disability and a case series. Isr J Psychiatry Relat Sci 2006;43:265–74.
32. Baer DM, Wolf MM, Risley TR. Some current dimensions of applied behavior analysis 1. J Appl Behav Anal 1968;1(1):91–7.
33. Eikeseth S, Klintwall L, Jahr E, et al. Outcome for children with autism receiving early and intensive behavioral intervention in mainstream preschool and kindergarten settings. Res Autism Spectr Disord 2012;6(2):829–35.
34. Sallows GO, Graupner TD. Intensive behavioral treatment for children with autism: Four-year outcome and predictors. Am J Ment Retard 2005;110(6): 417–38.
35. Smith T, Groen AD, Wynn JW. Randomized trial of intensive early intervention for children with pervasive developmental disorder. Am J Ment Retard 2000;105(4): 269–85.

36. Heyvaert M, Maes B, Van Den Noortgate W, et al. A multilevel meta-analysis of single-case and small-n research on interventions for reducing challenging behavior in persons with intellectual disabilities. Res Dev Disabil 2012;33(2): 766–80.

37. Harvey ST, Boer D, Meyer LH, et al. Updating a meta-analysis of intervention research with challenging behaviour: Treatment validity and standards of practice. J Intellect Dev Disabil 2009;34(1):67–80.

38. Brosnan J, Healy O. A review of behavioral interventions for the treatment of aggression in individuals with developmental disabilities. Res Dev Disabil 2011; 32(2):437–46.

39. Kahng S, Iwata BA, Lewin AB. Behavioral treatment of self-injury, 1964 to 2000. Am J Ment Retard 2002;107(3):212–21.

40. Lang R, Rispoli M, Machalicek W, et al. Treatment of elopement in individuals with developmental disabilities: A systematic review. Res Dev Disabil 2009;30(4): 670–81.

41. Doehring P, Reichow B, Palka T, et al. Behavioral approaches to managing severe problem behaviors in children with autism spectrum and related developmental disorders: A descriptive analysis. Child Adolesc Psychiatr Clin N Am 2014; 23(1):25–40.

42. Dawson G, Burner K. Behavioral interventions in children and adolescents with autism spectrum disorder: A review of recent findings. Curr Opin Pediatr 2011; 23(6):616–20.

43. Wong C, Odom S, Hume K, et al. Evidence-based practices for children, youth, and young adults with autism spectrum disorder: A comprehensive review. J Autism Dev Disord 2015;45(7):1951–66.

44. Center NA. National standards report. Randolph (MA): National Autism Center; 2009.

45. Neidert PL, Rooker GW, Bayles MW, et al. Functional analysis of problem behavior. Handbook of crisis intervention and developmental disabilities. Springer; 2013. p. 147–67.

46. Beavers GA, Iwata BA, Lerman DC. Thirty years of research on the functional analysis of problem behavior. J Appl Behav Anal 2013;46(1):1–21.

47. Hanley GP, Iwata BA, McCord BE. Functional analysis of problem behavior: a review. J Appl Behav Anal 2003;36(2):147–85.

48. Iwata BA, Pace GM, Dorsey MF, et al. The functions of self-injurious behavior: an experimental-epidemiological analysis. J Appl Behav Anal 1994;27(2):215–40.

49. Hagopian LP, Dozier CL, Rooker GW, et al. Assessment and treatment of severe problem behavior. In: Madden GJ, Dube WV, Hackenberg TD, et al, editors. APA handbook of behavior analysis, vol. 2. Washington, DC: American Psychological Association; 2013. p. 353–86. Translating Principles into Practice.

50. Kurtz PF, Boelter EW, Jarmolowicz DP, et al. An analysis of functional communication training as an empirically supported treatment for problem behavior displayed by individuals with intellectual disabilities. Res Dev Disabil 2011;32(6): 2935–42.

51. Chezan LC, Wolfe K, Drasgow E. A meta-analysis of functional communication training effects on problem behavior and alternative communicative responses. Focus Autism Other Dev Disabl 2018;33(4):195–205.

52. Greer BD, Fisher WW, Saini V, et al. Functional communication training during reinforcement schedule thinning: An analysis of 25 applications. J Appl Behav Anal 2016;49(1):105–21.

53. Hagopian LP, Fisher WW, Sullivan MT, et al. Effectiveness of functional communication training with and without extinction and punishment: a summary of 21 inpatient cases. J Appl Behav Anal 1998;31(2):211–35.

54. Rooker GW, Jessel J, Kurtz PF, et al. Functional communication training with and without alternative reinforcement and punishment: an analysis of 58 applications. J Appl Behav Anal 2013;46(4):708–22.

55. Carr JE, Severtson JM, Lepper TL. Noncontingent reinforcement is an empirically supported treatment for problem behavior exhibited by individuals with developmental disabilities. Res Dev Disabil 2009;30(1):44–57.

56. Richman DM, Barnard-Brak L, Grubb L, et al. Meta-analysis of noncontingent reinforcement effects on problem behavior. J Appl Behav Anal 2015;48(1): 131–52.

57. Lovaas OI. Behavioral treatment and normal educational and intellectual functioning in young autistic children. J Consult Clin Psychol 1987;55(1):3–9.

58. McEachin JJ, Smith T, Lovaas OI. Long-term outcome for children with autism who received early intensive behavioral treatment. Am J Ment Retard 1993;97: 359–72.

59. Alexander D. Prevention of mental retardation: Four decades of research. Ment Retard Dev Disabil Res Rev 1998;4(1):50–8.

60. Bailey DB Jr, Aytch LS, Odom SL, et al. Early intervention as we know it. Ment Retard Dev Disabil Res Rev 1999;5(1):11–20.

61. Ramey SL, Ramey CT. Early experience and early intervention for children "at risk"for developmental delay and mental retardation. Ment Retard Dev Disabil Res Rev 1999;5(1):1–10.

62. Kurtz PF, Chin MD, Huete JM, et al. Functional analysis and treatment of self-injurious behavior in young children:A summary of 30 cases. J Appl Behav Anal 2003;36(2):205–19.

63. Wacker DP, Berg WK, Harding JW, et al. Evaluation and long-term treatment of aberrant behavior displayed by young children with developmental disablities. J Dev Behav Pediatr 1998;19:260–6.

64. Derby KM, Wacker DP, Sasso G, et al. Brief functional assessment techniques to evaluate aberrant behavior in an outpatient setting: A summary of 79 cases. J Appl Behav Anal 1992;25(3):713–21.

65. Grindle CF, Kovshoff H, Hastings RP, et al. Parents' experiences of home-based applied behavior analysis programs for young children with autism. J Autism Dev Disord 2009;39(1):42–56.

66. Hanley GP, Heal NA, Tiger JH, et al. Evaluation of a classwide teaching program for developing preschool life skills. J Appl Behav Anal 2007;40(2):277–300.

67. Luczynski KC, Hanley GP. Prevention of problem behavior by teaching functional communication and self-control skills to preschoolers. J Appl Behav Anal 2013; 46(2):355–68.

68. Reeve CE, Carr EG. Prevention of severe behavior problems in children with developmental disorders. J Posit Behav Interv 2000;2(3):144.

69. Fahmie TA, Iwata BA, Mead SC. Within-subject analysis of a prevention strategy for problem behavior. J Appl Behav Anal 2016;49(4):915–26.

70. Fahmie TA, Macaskill AC, Kazemi E, et al. Prevention of the development of problem behavior: a laboratory model. J Appl Behav Anal 2018;51(1):25–39.

71. Hyman SL, Levy SE, Myers SM. Identification, evaluation, and management of children with autism spectrum disorder. Pediatrics 2020;145(1) [pii:e20193447].

72. Johnson CP, Myers SM. Identification and evaluation of children with autism spectrum disorders. Pediatrics 2007;120(5):1183–215.

73. Weissman L, Bridgemohan C, Augustyn M, et al. Autism spectrum disorder in children and adolescents: overview of management. UpToDate; 2018. p. 19.
74. Cui M, Graber JA, Metz A, et al. Parental indulgence, self-regulation, and young adults' behavioral and emotional problems. J Fam Stud 2019;25(3):233–49.
75. Fisher WW, Piazza CC, Bowman LG, et al. A preliminary evaluation of empirically derived consequences for the treatment of pica. J Appl Behav Anal 1994;27(3): 447–57.
76. LeClerc S, Easley D. Pharmacological therapies for autism spectrum disorder: a review. P T. 2015;40(6):389.
77. Almai AM, Hauptman AJ. Growing up with autism: Incorporating behavioral management and medication to manage self-injurious behavior. In: Hauptman A, Salpekar J, editors. Pediatric neuropsychiatry. Cham (Switzerland): Springer; 2019. p. 93–105.

Pediatric Prevention
Oral Health Care

Sara Kupzyk, PhD[a], Keith D. Allen, PhD[b],*

KEYWORDS

- Treatment of behavioral concerns • Anxiety/fear • Dental care • Oral health care

KEY POINTS

- A dental home may be difficult to establish when children demonstrate behavior management problems before or during treatment.
- Young children, those with separation anxiety, children with intellectual and developmental disabilities, children with toothaches, and those with caregivers who expect them to have behavior problems are more likely to have behavior management problems during dental care.
- Treatment of these behavior concerns should be developed with consideration of the underlying processes that produced them.
- Common elements of treatment include: graduated exposure, contingent reinforcement, modeling and prompting, distraction/relaxation, and cognitive behavior therapy.
- Having early, positive dental visits is useful for facilitating compliance and acceptance during routine visits.

The American Academy of Pediatric Dentistry recommends that primary care physicians and other professionals refer patients to establish a dental home no later than 12 months of age.[1] A dental home involves family-centered services for anticipatory guidance, education, routine care, individualized preventative health program, dietary counseling, and referral to dental specialists, and coordinated transition to adult providers. However, only 57% of families of children ages 2 to 5 receive advice about scheduling such visits.[2] Furthermore, 42% of children ages 2 to 11 have dental caries in the baby teeth, 23% of which go untreated.[3] Children who have a dental home are more likely to receive preventative care, require fewer dental treatments, and are less likely to have dental disease than those who do not have a dental home.

One potential challenge to establishing a dental home is behavioral concerns including noncompliance, aggression, and verbal protests that arise during dental

a Psychology, University of Nebraska, Omaha, NE, USA; b Psychology, Munroe-Meyer Institute for Genetics and Rehabilitation, University of Nebraska Medical Center, 985450 Nebraska Medical Center, Omaha, NE 68198, USA
* Corresponding author.
E-mail address: kdallen@unmc.edu

Pediatr Clin N Am 67 (2020) 513–524
https://doi.org/10.1016/j.pcl.2020.02.006   pediatric.theclinics.com
0031-3955/20/© 2020 Elsevier Inc. All rights reserved.

procedures. In fact, 44% of children ages 2 to 8 demonstrate negative acceptance on entering the treatment room and 23% show negative acceptance during dental examination.[4] Child characteristics associated with significantly more behavior management problems include:[4]

1. Being younger
2. Demonstrating anxiety when meeting new people
3. Having a toothache
4. Being diagnosed with an intellectual or developmental disability
5. Having guardians who expect that they will have negative behavior

For example, children that are younger do not fully understand the dental-care experience and are more likely to have developmentally appropriate stranger anxiety. The presence of a toothache is associated with pain and often requires more intensive procedures, which might be a negative experience that children continue to associate with going to dental appointments. In addition, children with autism spectrum disorder and other developmental and intellectual disabilities are more likely to present with problem behaviors during medical visits. These problematic behaviors are related to limited understanding, sensory sensitivities, and increased prevalence of anxiety in this population.[5,6] Children who have family members that have had negative dental experiences or report negative attitudes or fears related to dental care are also more likely to demonstrate behavior challenges.

Given the prevalence of behavior challenges, the American Academy of Pediatric Dentistry[7] outlined several behavior management strategies aimed to improve compliance with procedures, including: effective communication, modeling/use of visuals, voice control, distraction/brief breaks, memory restructuring, and parental presence. For more significant behavior concerns, the council outlined more invasive procedures, such as protective stabilization, sedation, and general anesthesia, all of which expose the patient to potential risks. To decrease the potential use of more invasive procedures, it is important for providers to (1) understand how behavior concerns related to dental visits might develop and continue, (2) describe strategies to prevent behavior concerns on initial referral, and (3) provide recommendations to intervene when such problems arise during dental visits.

UNDERSTANDING THE DEVELOPMENT AND MAINTENANCE OF BEHAVIOR MANAGEMENT CONCERNS

Behavior concerns during dental care are not surprising because routine medical procedures often involve stimuli associated with developmentally appropriate fears, such as unfamiliar settings and equipment, loud noises, strangers, separation, masks, the dark, and injections.[8,9] Although dental procedures are not a threat in any biologic sense,[10] the multiple fear-provoking features (eg, loud equipment, separation from parent, needles) make escape or avoidance logical and predictable. When children engage in such problematic behaviors, parents are also more likely to avoid dental routines.

Many fear behaviors are automatic responses elicited by natural triggers in the environment. Natural triggers are situations that automatically trigger fear and avoidance responses. These natural triggers may include loud noises from dental instruments, a prick on the gums, or scraping on the teeth. The automatic responses that are triggered can include mild, nonintrusive sweating, heart palpitations, shallow breathing, and nausea; and more disruptive behaviors, such flinching, blocking, fainting, and vomiting. Then, previously nonthreatening sights and sounds of the dental office environment (eg, the sight of a dental hygienist, the room where services are provided), through repeated pairing with unpleasant events, gradually become conditioned to trigger similar fear responses (**Fig. 1**). Over time, through even more pairings, more and more previously neutral stimuli (eg, the road in front of the office, similar looking buildings) can become conditioned to trigger fears and avoidance responses.

To compound the problems created by more and more dental situations triggering automatic fear and avoidance, those responses can also be strengthened and maintained by their consequences. That is, these emotional responses that often allow the individual to escape or avoid contact with feared events are reinforced, even though at times, the escape and avoidance are temporary at best. These behaviors can include a range of verbal (eg, crying, moaning, complaining) and physical protests (eg, pushing away, running away, biting, hitting). Unfortunately, here again because of repeated pairings with unpleasant events, previously neutral stimuli can acquire the ability to evoke noncompliant behaviors that, in the past, have produced escape or avoidance.

It is these escape and avoidance behaviors in particular that are at the heart of most noncompliance and have the potential to severely impact health outcomes by (1) creating risks of injury and increasing the use of restrictive means of gaining compliance (eg, sedation or restraint)[11]; (2) interfering with the completion of procedures; (3) deterring heath providers from a willingness to provide services, reducing access to care[12]; and (4) caregivers electing to avoid preventive or elective health care procedures because of the difficulties experienced when dealing with noncompliance. As a result of these complications, even a minor illness could create functional impairments, subsequent declines in health, and increased dependency on others for care.[13]

The conceptual analysis suggests that the focus of prevention and treatment of dental noncompliance should center on providing positive experiences with dental equipment, the office, and staff and extinction of the fear responses. Each is discussed in turn.

STRATEGIES FOR PREVENTING BEHAVIOR MANAGEMENT CONCERNS

From infancy, caregivers have an important role in supporting for their child's oral health. Providing information to families about appropriate oral hygiene practices

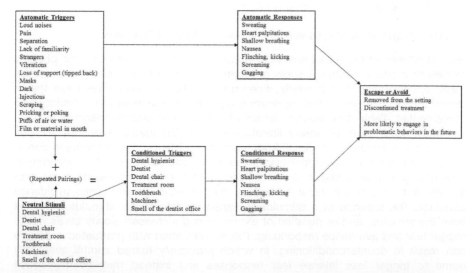

Fig. 1. Conditioning process of fear and avoidance behaviors during oral health care.

(eg, limiting juice/candy, regular brushing) can help to decrease the likelihood of toothaches and dental caries. The overall goal for prevention is to provide the child with positive experiences related to dental care and dental visits. In conversation with caregivers, practitioners can acknowledge that young children typically have some developmentally appropriate anxiety when attending the dentist. At the same time, it is important for caregivers to show confidence in the dental staff to help create an expectation for success in the child. To establish positive oral care routines practitioners can recommend that caregivers do the following[14]:

Instructions and Modeling
- Model appropriate brushing and flossing.
- Follow the same routine each day (eg, always brush in the morning and evening).
- Read books or watch videos that provide high-quality, developmentally appropriate information about oral care and visiting the dentist office.
- Request information when scheduling the initial appointment about what will happen (eg, will the child remain with the parent, how will the child be seated) and practice steps involved in the initial appointment with a doll/stuffed animal and with the child.

Reinforcement of appropriate oral care tasks
- Make positive statements about oral care.
- Offer choices (eg, would you like to use the red or blue toothbrush) to make the tasks more preferred.
- Provide positive attention and specific praise for good behavior (eg, playing nicely with toys in the waiting room, compliance with directions, opening mouth wide, following routines at home).

Graduated exposure
- If children show some anxiety or noncompliance with oral care:
  ○ Start small and increase the amount of time or number of teeth brushed/flossed if needed. The goal is for the child to have a good experience.
  ○ If needed, request to visit the dentist office briefly and leave on a good note to develop a positive connection between the dentist office and preferred attention, items, or activities.
  ○ Provide brief, planned breaks into routines.

INTERVENTIONS TO ADDRESS BEHAVIOR MANAGEMENT CONCERNS

Recent reviews of the broad empirical literature on treatment of fears and phobias related to medical treatment show graduated exposure to be the most common treatment approach.[15–17] Similarly, when problematic behaviors have been shown during dental care, graduated exposure is a primary component of treatment to be implemented. **Table 1** provides a sample of studies (also refer to Seligman and coworkers[18] for a more extensive literature review). Graduated exposure involves exposure to a hierarchy of stimuli from least to most feared that have been conditioned in the past to trigger fear responses and escape behavior. The hierarchy is arranged so that less salient stimuli (ie, stimuli that trigger less reaction) are presented first so that the initial exposures do not elicit fear or evoke avoidance behavior. The salience of a stimulus is varied by size of the stimulus, distance from the stimulus, and/or duration of exposure and increased slowly so as not to trigger fear and avoidance responding. Pairing relaxation with graduated exposure can result in counterconditioning, in which previously feared stimuli eventually come to trigger less intense fear responses and instead may even produce pleasant responses.

Table 1
Sample of experimental studies evaluating effects of treatments for dental nonadherence

Authors, Year, Ref.	Population	Study Design	Treatment Manual or Equivalent Description	Treatment Components	Treatment Outcomes
Allen & Wallace,[14] 2013	151 children, 2–9 y	Randomized, controlled, group design	Yes	NE	Tx group showed significantly fewer physical and vocal disruptive behaviors and lower need for restraint.
Boj & Davila,[19] 1989	28, 3–4 y	Matched control group design	Yes	VM	Tx group had higher heart rates and no differences in behavior or anxiety ratings.
Carter et al,[20] 2019	2 children, 10 and 18 y	Changing criterion	Yes	GE + Rfmt	The participants completed all steps in a simulated setting. Generalization data were collected for 1 child. He was able to complete the procedure.
Conyers et al,[21] 2004	6 adults	Multiple baseline across participants	Yes	GE + Rfmt + VM	VM was effective for 1 participant. All participants completed all 18 steps when desensitization package was implemented.
Cuvo et al,[22] 2010	5 children, 3–5 y	Multiple probe across participants	Yes	Dist + GE + Rfmt + VM + EE	Participants demonstrated compliance with the examinations and showed maintenance of responding.
Isong et al,[23] 2014	80 (20 in each of 4 groups), 7–17 y	Randomized controlled trial	No	VM vs Dist vs VM + Dist	No significant differences between groups (trend toward significance between control and distraction video goggles), although Dist and Dist + video modeling did show significant improvement within group.
Luscre & Center,[24] 1996	3 children, 6–9 y	Multiple baseline across participants	Yes	Dist + GE + IM + Rfmt	The participants completed all of the steps in an analog setting. Two completed 100% of steps in vivo, 1 completed 85% of steps.

(continued on next page)

Table 1
(continued)

Authors, Year, Ref.	Population	Study Design	Treatment Manual or Equivalent Description	Treatment Components	Treatment Outcomes
Orellana et al,[25] 2014	38 children and 34 adults	Preassessment, postassessment	Yes	GE + VM	There were significantly more components completed post-treatment. Ninety percent of the participants achieved 90%–100% steps completed.
Shahnavaz et al,[26] 2018	18 children, 7–15 y	Single-group, open-trial design	Yes	CBT	There was a significant change in self- and parent-perceived ability to manage dental care and reduction in proportion of participants diagnosed with dental anxiety.

Abbreviations: CBT, cognitive behavioral therapy; Dist, distraction/relaxation; EE, escape extinction; GE, graduated exposure; IM, in vivo modeling; NE, noncontingent escape; Rfmt, reinforcement; Tx, treatment; VM, video/picture modeling.

Graduated exposure can also be enhanced or strengthened by considering that noncompliant behaviors are often maintained by escape and avoidance of the planned medical routines. As a result, one might consider strategies that prevent escape or avoidance. However, these escape prevention procedures themselves are predicted to produce "bursts" of escape behavior, escalating in intensity, that further increase risks of harm to individuals and their caregivers or medical providers. Therefore, as an alternative, practitioners have developed approaches that emphasize reinforcement of cooperative behaviors (eg, sitting still), that are incompatible with noncompliance with medical routines. Gradually, the more fearful, or uncomfortable aspects of a medical routine are "faded in," but only after the individual has experienced success (ie, accessed reinforcement) for tolerating less threatening, less aversive conditions.

Gradual presentation of feared stimuli is most commonly accomplished by presenting the stimuli in the order in which they would be encountered in the actual procedure or reordering the stimuli into a fear hierarchy in which the steps that produce the least avoidance responses are presented first. A sample hierarchy is provided in **Box 1** based on those found in the literature.[22,27] In some cases, it may be necessary to revise the sequence of steps or add in substeps to promote compliance. Regardless of which approach is used, the steps in an exposure protocol are sequenced based on dimensions, such as duration of exposure to the stimulus, size of the stimulus, or distance from a stimulus.[16] For example, the number of minutes, size of a device/material/medication, and distance to device/materials/equipment can be gradually increased.

Box 1
Sample fear hierarchy

1. Enter the waiting room

2. Sit in waiting room for 5 minutes

3. Walk to dental chair with parent

4. Sit in dental chair

5. Sit in dental chair for 5 minutes

6. Open mouth while sitting in chair

7. Keep mouth open while assistant places tool in mouth

8. Keep mouth open while assistant counts teeth

9. Keep mouth open for assistant to remove plaque from teeth (gradually increase number of teeth completed)

10. Keep mouth open while assistant brushes teeth

11. Put water in mouth

12. Spit water out of mouth into cup

13. Place apron over shoulders

14. Open mouth

15. Bite down and hold teeth together for radiograph

16. Open mouth to remove

17. Sit in chair for dentist

18. Open mouth for dentist

19. Walk to waiting room

The core mechanism of change in graduated exposure is the disruption of the association between triggers and fear responses resulting, hypothetically, in a process called "extinction." The addition of a relaxation response during the exposures focuses additionally on undoing the previous conditioning. Here, the point of emphasis is on the individual being relaxed before the presentation of the feared stimuli and then maintaining relaxation during the presentations. This particular form of graduated exposure is commonly called systematic desensitization.[28] In contrast, the addition of a positive consequence for compliance and acceptance or other desired behaviors focuses on reinforcement of calm and compliant behaviors. Here, the point of emphasis is on delivering reinforcement after the presentation of the fear stimuli contingent on the individual exhibiting cooperative behaviors.

Although graduated exposure seems to be one of the most important components of treatment,[29] it is typically combined with other strategies in a treatment package to address behavior management concerns. A description of each strategy is provided in **Table 2**. Each of these components is designed to reduce the probability of problem behaviors occurring from the outset and/or to reinforce more appropriate responding. Nevertheless, it is important to consider how one will respond to noncompliance when it does occur. Responses to noncompliance have typically involved (1) physically blocking escape attempts and guiding compliance; (2) taking brief breaks from trials, ignoring the problem behavior, and then continuing exposure trials (escape permitted

Table 2
Strategies to reduce the probability of behavior concerns and increase compliance with dental routines, visits, and procedures

Strategy	Description
Graduated exposure	The child is exposed to a hierarchy of stimuli from least to most feared that have been conditioned in the past to elicit fear responses and escape behavior. The hierarchy is arranged so that less salient stimuli are presented first so that the initial exposures do not elicit fear or evoke avoidance behavior.
Contingent reinforcement	A reinforcer (eg, preferred activity, item, break, or token that can be exchanged) is given to the child for meeting specific expectations (eg, compliance, opening mouth for a certain amount of time, completing a step). The expectations must be reasonable and gradually increased so that the child can receive the reinforcement. Potential reinforcers are identified through caregiver interviews or preference assessments.
Modeling and prompting	An in vivo model, video, pictures, or stories are used to demonstrate the step/what will happen for the child. For example, the provider might tell and show the child what will happen before administering the procedure.
Distraction/relaxation	The child is given access to preferred activities or taught relaxation responses to try to elicit positive responses to counter the fear response.
Noncontingent escape	The child is given brief breaks at regular time intervals during the procedure.
Cognitive behavior therapy	Therapy focused on understanding the relationship between feelings, thinking, and behavior to improve functioning. Patients are taught how to identify cognitive distortions and develop more realistic thoughts and engage in more adaptive behaviors.

Box 2
Summary of recommendations

Preventing the need for treatment of noncompliance with medical/dental routines
1. Find medical and dental professionals experienced and comfortable with individuals with managing behavioral concerns and working with children with disabilities
2. Parents/caregivers get permission to plan multiple 10-minute "field trips" to medical/dental clinic
3. Providers are asked to approve visit with only relaxing and reinforcing activities
4. Parents request no exposure to masks, gowns, gloves, or typical medical/dental instruments
5. Parents bring preferred toys, activities, edibles with them
6. Emphasis is ending visit while individual is relaxed and enjoying themselves
7. Subsequent trips might include gradual exposure to stimuli (not those that already are conditioned as aversive)

Preparation for treatment of medical/dental noncompliance
1. Conduct a task analysis
2. Develop a fear hierarchy
3. Conduct no treatment exposures; observe the intensity of behavior, features of most salient stimuli (eg, distance, size, duration, or intensity of exposure), and how far the client is able to progress
4. Revise the task analysis to include any necessary substeps
5. Conduct a preference assessment to identify tangible items and passive activities that can be used as reinforcers delivered contingent on desired calm, "coping" behaviors after each exposure

Treatment of medical/dental noncompliance
1. Provide noncontingent access to some preferred items to distract/relax the individual before the exposures begin
2. Use in vivo modeling of appropriate behavior by a parent or caregiver of appropriate behavior before or during graduated exposures
3. Begin graduated exposure (core component of treatment) and provide reinforcement for compliance
4. Progress to the next step when the individual has been compliant with the current step and appears relaxed
5. Back up to easier steps if necessary to establish success
6. Plan for how to handle disruptive behavior and determine when escape extinction might be needed based on treatment necessity (Note: researchers have typically had good success without escape extinction, but this may require a more gradual approach to exposures that lengthens the course of treatment)

---

for brief periods); or (3) ending exposure trials when problems occurred (escape permitted that day). Although the latter two approaches offer only temporary escape (because exposure trials ultimately begin again), even temporary escape or avoidance can help maintain fear and noncompliance.[14] Regardless of the approach taken, these procedures are rarely used in isolation, but were used in combination with efforts to reduce the probability of noncompliance while reinforcing incompatible alternatives.

SUMMARY

Step-by-step practice recommendations for preventing the need for treatment of noncompliance with medical/dental routines, preparing for treatment of noncompliance, and implementing treatment of noncompliance are included in **Box 2**. Medical providers are a vital point of contact for families and can aid in the development of a dental home to decrease the likelihood of dental caries and more significant dental and related health problems. Providers should be aware of predictors related to behavior management concerns during dental care, how behavior concerns typically develop, and strategies to prevent and intervene to address such concerns. The recommendations provided can help families to develop a course of action to address behavioral concerns; however, when concerns are clinically significant, families are referred to appropriate behavioral health providers for more intensive intervention.

Given that the process of graduated exposure treatment packages is time-consuming, they may initially seem unattractive to providers because most are paid by procedure as opposed to time spent with patients. However, the time spent on procedures to increase compliance (as early as possible) is likely to lead to improved health outcomes over time (eg, fewer dental treatment and less dental disease) and fewer intensive and more costly procedures (eg, surgery, sedation, restraint). Additional support and advocacy for reimbursement of procedures to increase compliance with dental care are needed. In addition, providers would benefit from more extensive training in the use of behavior management strategies. Such trainings can be incorporated into courses or internship requirements to better prepare dental providers to prevent and intervene to address problematic behaviors.[30] Lastly, innovative approaches, such as interactive Internet-based programs[26] or virtual reality treatments,[31] should be further explored because these methods may reduce the time needed for treatment in the dental office, thus decreasing provider time spent.

DISCLOSURE

The authors have nothing to disclose.

REFERENCES

1. AAPD Pediatric Oral Health Research and Policy Center. Snapshot of America's children. 2018. Available at: https://www.aapd.org/assets/1/7/Childs_Snapshot_2018_web_version.pdf. Accessed June 20, 2019.
2. American Academy of Pediatric Dentistry, Council on Clinical Affairs. Policy on the dental home. 2018. Available at: https://www.aapd.org/media/policies_guidelines/p_dentalhome.pdf. Accessed June 20, 2019.
3. National Institute of Dental and Craniofacial Research. National Health and Nutrition Examination Survey (NHANES). 2018. Available at: https://www.nidcr.nih.gov/research/data-statistics/dental-caries/children. Accessed June 22, 2019.
4. Sharma A, Kumar D, Anand A, et al. Factors predicting behavior management problems during initial dental examination in children aged 2 to 8 years. Int J Clin Pediatr Dent 2017;10(1):5–9.
5. Pruijssers AC, van Meijel B, Maaskant M, et al. The relationship between challenging behaviour and anxiety in adults with intellectual disabilities: a literature review. J Intellect Disabil Res 2014;58:162–71.
6. Fallea A, Zuccarello R, Cali F. Dental anxiety in patients with borderline intellectual functioning and patients with intellectual disabilities. BMC Oral Health 2016;16:114–20.
7. American Academy of Pediatric Dentistry, Council on Clinical Affairs. Behavior guidance for the pediatric dental patient. Reference manual. 2015;40(6). Available at: https://www.aapd.org/globalassets/media/policies_guidelines/bp_behavguide.pdf. Accessed June 22, 2019.
8. Gullone E. The development of normal fear: a century of research. Clin Psychol Rev 2005;20:429–51.
9. Silverman WK. Fears and phobias. In: Koocher G, la Greca A, editors. The parents guide to psychological first aid. Oxford (England): University Press; 2011. p. 231–8.

10. Muehlhan M, Lueken U, Wittchen H, et al. The scanner as a stressor: evidence from subjective and neuroendocrine stress parameters in the time course of a functional magnetic resonance imaging session. Int J Psychophysiol 2011;79: 118–26.
11. Camoin A, Dany L, Tardieu C, et al. Ethical issues and dentists' practices with children with intellectual disability: a qualitative inquiry into a local French health network. Disabil Health J 2018;11:412–9.
12. Lennox N, Kerr M. Primary health care and people with an intellectual disability: the evidence base. J Intellect Disabil Res 1997;41:365–72.
13. Rimmer JH. Health promotion for people with disabilities: emerging paradigm shift from disability prevention to prevention of secondary conditions. Phys Ther 1999;79:495–502.
14. Allen KD, Wallace DW. Effectiveness of using noncontingent escape for general behavior management in a pediatric dental clinic. J Appl Behav Anal 2013;46: 723–37.
15. Davis TE, Ollendick TH. Empirically supported treatments for specific phobia in children: do efficacious treatments address the components of a phobic response? Clin Psychol Sci Pract 2005;12:144–60.
16. Jennett HK, Hagopian LP. Identifying empirically supported treatments for phobic avoidance in individuals with intellectual disabilities. Behav Ther 2008;39:151–61.
17. Lydon S, Healy O, O'Callaghan O, et al. A systematic review of the treatment of fears and phobias among children with autism spectrum disorders. Rev J Autism Dev Disord 2015;2:141–54.
18. Seligman LD, Hovey JD, Chacon K, et al. Dental anxiety: an understudied problem in youth. Clin Psychol Rev 2017;55:25–40.
19. Boj JR, Davila JM. A study of behavior modification for developmentally disabled children. J Dent Child 1989;56:452–7.
20. Carter L, Harper JM, Luiselli JK. Dental desensitization for students with autism spectrum disorder through graduated exposure, reinforcement, and reinforcement-fading. J Dev Phys Disabil 2019;31:161–70.
21. Conyers C, Miltenberger RG, Peterson B, et al. An evaluation of an in vivo desensitization and video modeling to increase compliance with dental procedures in persons with mental retardation. J Appl Behav Anal 2004;37:233–8.
22. Cuvo AJ, Godard A, Huckfeldt R, et al. Training children with autism spectrum disorders to be compliant with an oral assessment. Res Autism Spectr Disord 2010;4:681–96.
23. Isong IA, Rao SR, Holifield C, et al. Addressing dental fear in children with autism spectrum disorders: a randomized controlled pilot using electronic screen media. Clin Pediatr 2014;53:230–7.
24. Luscre DM, Center DB. Procedures for reducing dental fear in children with autism. J Autism Dev Disord 1996;26:547–56.
25. Orellana LM, Martinez-Sanchis S, Silvestre FJ. Training adults and children with an autism spectrum disorder to be compliant with a clinical dental assessment using a TEACCH-based approach. J Autism Dev Disord 2014;44:776–85.
26. Shahnavaz S, Hedman-Lagerlöf E, Hasselblad T, et al. Internet-based cognitive behavioral therapy for children and adolescents with dental anxiety: open trial. J Med Internet Res 2018;20(1):e12.
27. Altabet SC. Decreasing dental resistance among individuals with severe and profound mental retardation. J Dev Phys Disabil 2002;14:297–305.
28. King NJ, Muris P, Ollendick TH. Childhood fears and phobias: assessment and treatment. Child Adolesc Ment Health 2005;10:50–6.

29. Kupzyk S, Allen KD. A review of strategies to increase comfort and compliance with medical/dental routines in persons with intellectual and developmental disabilities. J Dev Phys Disabil 2019;31(2):231–49.
30. Graudins MM, Rehfeldt RA, DeMattei R, et al. Exploring the efficacy of behavioral skills training to teach basic behavior analytic techniques to oral care providers. Res Autism Spectr Disord 2012;6:978–87.
31. Gujjar KR, van Wijk A, Kumar R, et al. Efficacy of virtual reality exposure therapy for the treatment of dental phobia in adults: a randomized controlled trial. J Anxiety Disord 2019;62:100–8.

Autism Spectrum Disorder
Characteristics, Associated Behaviors, and Early Intervention

Tiffany Kodak, PhD, BCBA-D[a],*, Samantha Bergmann, PhD, BCBA-D[b]

KEYWORDS

- ASD • Autism spectrum disorder • Early intervention • Early behavioral intervention
- Social skills • Language • Adaptive behavior

KEY POINTS

- A child diagnosed with autism spectrum disorder (ASD) is likely to have a range of behavioral deficits and excesses to address in intervention.
- Behavioral deficits may include social communication, language development, and adaptive skills, and behavioral excesses may include forms of problem behavior.
- Interventions based on principles of applied behavior analysis (ABA) can effectively reduce social skills deficits following training.
- Approaches to language development and communication based on ABA incorporate a functional approach to language and can effectively increase verbal and nonverbal communication skills.
- Teaching strategies based on ABA can be used to teach adaptive skills, like daily living skills, to help individuals with ASD acquire more independence.

Autism spectrum disorder (ASD) is a neurodevelopmental disorder characterized by deficits in social communication and social interaction and the presence of restricted, repetitive patterns of behavior, interests, or activities present during early periods of development that negatively impact social, occupational, or other domains.[1] Different combinations and ranges of behavioral deficits and excesses are associated with an ASD diagnosis; therefore, ASD can affect individuals along a continuum of severity.[1] The cause of ASD is unknown, but research supports genetic and environmental factors.[2] One in every 59 children has a diagnosis of ASD,[3] and ASD is 4 times as likely to occur in male than female individuals.[4] ASD affects individuals across racial, ethnic, and socioeconomic boundaries and has a high likelihood of occurring with another

[a] Department of Psychology, Marquette University, 525 North 6th Street, Milwaukee, WI 53203, USA; [b] Department of Behavior Analysis, University of North Texas, 1155 Union Circle #310919, Denton, TX 76203-5017, USA
* Corresponding author.
E-mail address: tiffany.kodak@marquette.edu

Pediatr Clin N Am 67 (2020) 525–535
https://doi.org/10.1016/j.pcl.2020.02.007
0031-3955/20/© 2020 Elsevier Inc. All rights reserved.

developmental disorder (ie, 83%) or psychiatric disorder (ie, 10%).[4] The average age of diagnosis is 5 years; however, early warning signs can be observed in infancy.[5] Longitudinal studies of infants at risk for developing ASD reported several behaviors, including poor eye contact, lack of visual tracking, no orientation to name, few imitation skills, lack of social interest, and limited language.[6,7]

Early social skills begin to emerge at very young ages in children of typical development, but children with ASD often require targeted interventions to learn these foundational skills (eg, joint attention, social referencing, social engagement).[8] Social skills are necessary for children to adapt to their environment and interact appropriately with others. Deficits in social skills may create limited relationships with peers and family members, likely straining familial relationships.[9] Thus, early intervention should emphasize building skills for success in social opportunities like vocal communication.

An impairment in vocal language is not required for a diagnosis of ASD; however, a diagnosis may specify if the individual has an accompanying language impairment.[1] The acquisition of "useful language" by 2 years old is the strongest predictor of positive developmental trajectories,[10] and vocal language is one of the strongest predictors of positive long-term outcomes for children with ASD.[11] The acquisition of speech by 5 or 6 years of age is associated with greater academic achievement and social independence and competence.[11]

In addition to deficits in social communication and interaction, approximately one-third of children with ASD have deficient adaptive or daily living skills.[3] This domain is not directly related to the core features of ASD; nevertheless, many individuals with ASD require intervention to acquire adaptive skills (eg, toileting, grooming).[9,12] Deficits in adaptive skills may further limit the opportunities for social involvement in education and community settings due to issues with safety (eg, disrobing in public), availability of proper resources (eg, family restrooms), or social stigmatization. Individuals with ASD are more likely than their peers to remain dependent on others for care throughout the life span.[12] Deficits in adaptive skills and decreased independence require that parents and caregivers provide more assistance to children with ASD to complete tasks, which may limit the caregivers' ability to spend time with others, work outside of the home, and develop and maintain their interpersonal relationships.[9] Therefore, it is important to address adaptive skill deficits in early intervention as well.

Problem behavior, although not one of the core diagnostic features of ASD, is one of the main reasons for referral to services[5] and a source of parental or caregiver stress and concern.[13] Broadly defined, problem behavior is that which is not socially acceptable, may be physically dangerous, and negatively impacts functioning (eg, aggression, self-injurious behavior, tantrums, property destruction, elopement).[14] Children with ASD are more likely than children with an intellectual disability, a psychiatric disorder, or typical development to engage in problem behavior.[15,16] Estimates of the proportion of individuals with ASD who engage in at least one type of problem behavior vary widely, with some published studies reporting prevalence estimates as low as 8% or 25%[9] and as high as 94%.[14,15] In general, problem behavior is associated with poorer outcomes overall and is the factor most likely to lead to residential placement,[16] and the use of pharmacotherapy (eg, antipsychotics).[15]

Problem behavior may affect skill development in social communication and social interaction, a core deficit of ASD.[13] Individuals with ASD, especially those who engage in problem behavior, are more likely than typically developing peers to experience low rates of peer acceptance and high rates of peer rejection.[13] Problem behavior can lead to increased isolation, interfere with educational and therapeutic interventions, and limit participation in social and community activities because of safety concerns.[16]

Problem behavior is likely to persist and increase in frequency and severity and is unlikely to be resolved without intervention.[13] As children develop physically, intervention can become more difficult and dangerous.[15] Therefore, early intervention to reduce problem behavior and replace it with functional skills is crucial (for more detailed information on problem behavior, see the article by Patricia F. Kurtz and colleagues' article, "Behavioral Approaches to Assessment and Early Intervention for Severe Problem Behavior in Intellectual and Developmental Disabilities," elsewhere in this issue).

Given the breadth and depth of behavioral deficits and excesses associated with ASD, it may be no surprise to learn that the economic costs of ASD are staggering. In the United States, estimated annual costs for children with ASD range from $11.5 billion to $60.9 billion.[4] These costs include medical care, loss of parental wages, and special education or intervention.[4] Over one's lifetime, the costs of caring for an individual with ASD can exceed $2 million.[17] Nevertheless, the reported economic costs of ASD may not adequately describe the extent of public health costs because collateral costs like parental or familial stress are not included.[17]

PREVENTION AND EARLY INTERVENTION

The increasing prevalence of ASD and substantial economic and collateral costs at the individual, familial, and societal levels necessitate attention to interventions that could serve to prevent the development or exacerbation of behaviors associated with ASD. A child with ASD will likely have needs in several areas, including social communication and interaction, vocal language, adaptive skills, and problem behavior. Strategies to prevent and intervene early on behavioral excesses and deficits associated with ASD can reduce the child's level of impairment in adaptive, educational, and behavioral skills. There is extensive empirical support for early intervention based on the principles of applied behavior analysis (ABA), leading to mandated insurance coverage for interventions for children with ASD in 49 states and the District of Columbia.[18] The most significant gains are likely to occur if a child begins intervention before 5 years of age[14]; however, ABA interventions are effective across the life span.[19]

There are many evidence-based ABA practices to address behavioral deficits and excesses associated with ASD and related disorders.[19] We describe several evidence-based methods for developing early social skills, increasing communication, and establishing independence in functional life skills.

Behavioral Intervention to Establish Early Social Skills

Social and communication skills are critical behaviors to acquire in early childhood for an improved developmental trajectory and acquisition of more complex skills.[5] Early social communication skills (ESCS), including eye contact, coordinated eye gaze shifting, joint attention, social referencing, and social orienting, often emerge via everyday interactions throughout the first 24 months.[5,8] Although these skills are thought to be critical for development of more advanced social skills and predict success in academic, social, and adaptive contexts, additional research on ESCS with an emphasis on identifying pivotal skills and components of intervention that are most likely to lead to improvements.[9] Despite the need for additional research, existing evidence supports the use of ABA to assess, teach, and maintain these important skills.[5] Strategies described as follows have been shown to increase ESCS with very young children, including infants.[5] The information that follows focuses primarily on joint attention; however, common techniques, such as providing reinforcers (ie, a consequence provided following a behavior makes it more likely to occur under similar circumstances in the future), prompting (ie, providing assistance to get the behavior to occur and removing the assistance systematically until the child engages in the behavior independently), and arranging motivating conditions (ie, events that occur before a behavior that make a behavior more likely and make a consequence more effective) can be applied to teach many ESCS.

Joint attention is the coordination or sharing of attention between 2 people and an object or event.[20] Joint attention begins as a gaze shift (ie, child looks from an interesting item or event to a familiar person and then back to the item) and progresses to include combinations of eye gaze shift, vocalizations, and gestures (eg, pointing, reaching, showing object to a person).[21] Joint attention typically develops between the ages of 9 and 15 months, and is crucial to the development of language.[22] Children with ASD often have delayed or impaired joint attention.[23] In fact, delayed or deficient joint attention is one of the behaviors used for early diagnosis of ASD.[21] The acquisition of joint attention skills can be used to evaluate a child's progress in an early intervention program.[24] Furthermore, joint attention deficits have been associated with difficulties acquiring vocal language and developing social competence.[21,23] For these reasons, joint attention skills are targeted in early intervention programs for children with ASD.

Joint attention is typically divided into 2 categories: (1) responding to joint attention and (2) initiating joint attention.[25] Both categories of joint attention begin with an interesting or novel item or activity in the environment (ie, a motivating condition), but they differ in terms of who attends to the interesting situation and seeks to share the experience with another person. A defining feature of joint attention responses and initiations is that the consequence for responding is social in nature because they produce shared attention to an item or activity (eg, both individuals looking at the item, an adult reaction to the item).

In a joint attention response, an adult or peer begins the interaction by pointing to, looking at, or gesturing toward an item or object in the child's environment.[25] After this gesture (perhaps with an accompanying vocalization like "Look!"), the child shifts his or her gaze (ie, looks from the person to the item and back to the person) and may comment on the item or activity. Then, the adult or peer makes a comment to the child or provides another social interaction like smiles or attention. For example, when walking with her child in the neighborhood, a mother spots a deer in a nearby yard, which is an unusual sight. The mother says, "Wow! Look over there!" and points to the deer. Her toddler looks from her to the deer and then back to her. The mother says, "It's a treat to see a deer here!" and smiles at her toddler.

In a joint attention initiation, the child engages in behavior to direct the adult's attention to the same item or activity.[25] For example, a child sees a deer, turns to her mother, and says "Mommy, look!" while turning her gaze back to the deer. The mother shifts her gaze to the location of the deer, says, "Wow! The deer is so pretty!" and turns back to her daughter to share her delight. Thus, the child recruits her mother's attention to share the experience, and the mother's attention is the reinforcer for the joint attention initiation.

Although children with ASD may require intervention for both types of joint attention, joint attention initiation is often impaired to a greater degree and less likely to emerge without targeted intervention.[24] Joint attention responses may occur because following an adult's directions has been previously taught and reinforced with preferred items.[21] In comparison, joint attention initiations may be conceptualized as a mand (ie, request; described later in this article) for shared attention or experiences rather than the receipt of an item or information.[21,26] If social attention and reactions of others are not effective reinforcers (ie, do not make a behavior more likely to occur in the future) for a child with ASD, then it is unlikely that the child will initiate an interaction that is purely social in nature (ie, joint attention initiations). Core deficits related to social communication and social awareness observed in children with ASD could help explain difficulties acquiring joint attention without intervention.

Taylor and Hoch[26] taught children with ASD to respond to and initiate joint attention within an early intervention program by carefully arranging motivating situations to create conditions for shared interest. Motivating situations were rotated often and included novel toys, altering the appearance of toys (eg, placing a clown wig on a toy horse), placing items in unusual locations or positions (eg, a bicycle turned upside down). The consequence for joint attention initiations and responses were social interest and not access to an item. Following intervention, children with ASD increased both joint attention responses and initiations. Joint attention is only one social skill, albeit a critically important one, that can be impaired in children with ASD and should be addressed with ABA treatment. When a child with ASD responds to and initiates joint attention with familiar people in their lives, this can be the beginning of building a shared social experience and interactive communication.[26]

Behavioral Intervention to Increase Communication

Interventions based on ABA are not the only option to address language deficits for children with ASD. However, an ABA-based approach to language development is unique to other forms of therapy in that it prioritizes the function of language, rather than the topography (ie, the specific words) or form, and examines the consequences produced by language. Other approaches to language acquisition (eg, linguistics) may assume that once a child acquires a word, that word is a representation or symbol of the item, and he or she will be able to use that word whenever appropriate. In contrast, an ABA-based approach to language (also called verbal behavior or the verbal behavior approach), with a focus on function, operates under the assumption that the child needs to learn to use that word under a variety of conditions; this is called functional independence.

Communication intervention based on ABA means that a practitioner carefully determines under which conditions language is (or is not) occurring and designs intervention to increase language based on the conditions and reinforcers. Assessments of and interventions for language are based on the verbal operants, the unit of language outlined by Skinner,[27] and the technical terms in this taxonomy are described as follows with a focus on the stimuli that occur before and following language. Skinner outlined 4 elementary verbal operants: the echoic, mand, tact, and intraverbal, which are commonly targeted in early intervention. Early intervention may focus on teaching communication through vocalizations, manual signs, or picture exchange systems.

The *echoic* is a verbal operant that matches, or closely approximates, the spoken or signed word that comes before it. The echoic is maintained or increased by a generalized reinforcer that follows it (eg, praise, hugs, tickles, and smiles). For example, a mother says, "airplane," the child repeats, "airplane," and the mother says, "so good!" while tickling her child. A proportion of early parent and child interactions attempt to establish echoic behavior, such as when a mother tries to get her young child to say "dada" when dad is not present. Echoic behavior can be used to establish other verbal operants (described as follows), because an adult can have the child imitate or repeat the vocalization in novel contexts.

The *mand* is a verbal operant that is a request for items, activities, or information that occurs under motivating conditions (eg, deprivation, aversive stimulation) that make these consequences reinforcers. The mand specifies its reinforcer, meaning that the vocalizations included in the response are typically associated with the consequence.

For example, the mand, "I want the airplane," indicates that giving the toy airplane to the child will reinforce (ie, strengthen) that response. Mands occur when a person is present who can provide the reinforcers. Mands are the verbal operant with the greatest benefit to the speaker, because mands allow the child to communicate to gain access to wants and needs in his or her environment.[28] Thus, mands are typically one of the first verbal operants taught in early intervention.

Initially, mands for items are targeted in early intervention by identifying preferred items (eg, toys, activities) and providing access to the items following targeted vocalizations, signs, or picture exchanges. When teaching mands, the therapist should arrange for a motivating condition like deprivation (eg, putting a favorite toy away for a period), as these are the environmental conditions that should lead to a mand in any setting. Mand training may establish initial sounds (eg,/oo/for cookie) or single-word mands (eg, cookie, music) with the complexity of the mand increasing over time, such as requiring full sentences (eg, "May I have a cookie, please?" "Will you sing a song?"). In addition to accessing toys and activities, mands also help children acquire more control over their environment. Mand training can be used to teach a child to change or remove someone or something that is aversive. For example, a therapist may teach a child who cries when loud music is played near him to say, "Please turn it down." For more on replacing problem behavior with appropriate behavior see the article by Patricia F. Kurtz and colleagues' article, "Behavioral Approaches to Assessment and Early Intervention for Severe Problem Behavior in Intellectual and Developmental Disabilities," elsewhere in this issue.

Subsequent training targets mands for information, and the training context is designed to establish the receipt of information as a reinforcer. Early mand for information training might begin by hiding a child's favorite toy. When the child looks for the toy but cannot find it, training the mand for information occurs (eg, "Where is my fire truck?"). Immediately following the mand, the therapist gives the child the information that can be used to find the item (eg, "Your fire truck is under the couch"). Information on the whereabouts of the toy allows the child to find and play with the toy. Once learned, additional training could include mands for information about other people, items, and activities in their environment.

The *tact* is a verbal operant that is like a label of a nonverbal stimulus (eg, an object in the environment, a picture, a sound, a flavor) that produces generalized reinforcers (eg, praise, attention, tickles). For example, a child looks up at the sky and says, "Airplane" as an airplane zooms overhead, and the adult provides social interaction like saying, "Wow! That is a really big plane." Tacts permit children to speak about the environment around them and communicate or share the environment with others. A therapist might teach a child to tact a shoe by showing the child a variety of 2-dimensional and 3-dimensional shoes and providing a prompt (eg, "Say, shoe") until the child independently tacts different examples of shoes. The use of prompts and prompt fading are highly effective in teaching verbal operants to children with ASD, and this type of training can rapidly expand a child's contact and familiarity with objects in his or her environment.[28]

The *intraverbal* is a verbal operant that follows a verbal stimulus (eg, a question, statement), but, unlike the echoic, the intraverbal does not match the preceding verbal stimulus. For example, a peer may ask, "What is your favorite toy," the child replies "airplane," and the peer provides social interaction like "I like planes, too." In typical language development, a child acquires quite a few mands and tacts before early intraverbal behavior emerges.[28] Thus, in early intervention, intraverbal training with children with ASD occurs after establishing some echoics, mands, and tacts, and the acquisition of intraverbal behavior is facilitated when relevant mands and tacts are learned first. For example, the child should be able to tact food and the action of eating before being taught intraverbal responses to a question like "What do you eat?"

Early intraverbals are generally simpler and may involve teaching fill-in-the-blank statements during interactive activities like games and songs. For example, if siblings are going to race toy cars on a track, the brother may say, "ready, set..." and wait for the sister with ASD to say, "go" before starting the race. Parents may also help to establish early intraverbal behavior by singing songs with their child with ASD and allowing the child to fill in the missing words (eg, "Old McDonald had a..."). Therapists establish other types of intraverbals that increase in complexity during early intervention, such as teaching answers to a variety of wh- (eg, what, who, where, when, and why) questions.

Intraverbals are one of the most important verbal operants because they form the basis for social interactions with others, conversations, and the development of friendships. Language without a robust intraverbal repertoire that includes appropriate responses to questions that further the conversation can limit social development.[29] In other words, it would be difficult to have a complete and meaningful conversation composed of only echoics, mands, and tacts.[29] Therefore, a particularly lengthy period of intervention is allocated to intraverbal training. Although some research suggests a sequence of simple to more complex intraverbals may be acquired by typically developing children and children with ASD,[29] considerably more research is necessary to establish prerequisite skills for specific types of intraverbal training and to understand better how to establish this critical but complex verbal operant in children with ASD.

Behavioral Intervention to Establish Independent Living Skills

Children with ASD often have deficits in adaptive skills that reduce independence. For example, children with ASD may not complete daily hygiene routines, such as getting dressed, brushing teeth, and taking a shower. The level of support that an individual with ASD requires to complete activities of daily living is negatively correlated with greater integration into society and independent living arrangements.[9] Further, many young children with ASD are not toilet trained.[30] Reliance on supports from an adult to complete daily hygiene routines (eg, toileting) may increases a child's likelihood of abuse, which is especially concerning given that rates of sexual abuse in children with intellectual disabilities are 4 times that of typically developing children.[31] Children who are not independent with daily living skills may miss out on social and educational opportunities, such as children who are unable to play dress up with peers because they cannot dress themselves.

Because of their importance, adaptive and independent living skills are often targeted in early intervention. Training of these skills typically occurs in several steps. The first step of intervention is to create a *task analysis*, which involves generating a step-by-step list of the behavior chain (ie, sequence of behaviors) that an individual engages in when completing the task (see **Table 1** for an example). ABA practitioners may engage in the behavior chain themselves or watch an expert perform the skill while writing down the sequence of steps to create task analyses. Task analyses should be flexible with steps that can be combined if the child moves through them quickly, broken down further if a child needs additional support and practice, or adjusted to reflect how the child or the child's family completes the task. For example, the handwashing task analysis (see **Table 1**) would be modified if the family gets soap and rubs their dry hands together before wetting their hands.

After completing the task analysis, the next step is to identify an intervention to teach the child with ASD to complete the adaptive task. Several empirically validated

Table 1
Example task analysis for handwashing

Step	Behavior
1	Move stool in front of sink
2	Step onto stool
3	Turn on water (hot and cold faucet handles)
4	Place both hands under water
5	Turn off water
6	Grab soap
7	Put soap in hand
8	Rub hands together
9	Rub top of one hand
10	Rub top of other hand
11	Place both hands under water
12	Rinse hands until soap is gone
13	Turn off water (hot and cold faucet handles)
14	Grab towel
15	Dry hands

training procedures have been used to teach children and adults with ASD and other developmental disabilities to successfully engage in behavior chains.[30] Four of those training procedures are forward chaining, backward chaining, total-task presentation, and activity schedules. *Forward chaining* involves teaching the very first step in the behavior chain and then adding steps one at a time. For example, the first step in the handwashing task analysis in **Table 1** is moving the stool in front of the sink. Initially, the child would need to complete this step independently before accessing a reinforcer (eg, brief playtime on a tablet). Once the child is consistently performing Step 1, then Step 2 (ie, step onto stool) would be added. Thus, the child would need to perform Steps 1 and 2 before accessing the reinforcer. This sequence of adding a step once earlier steps are completed independently continues until the child can execute all steps in the behavior chain.

Backward chaining also involves teaching one step and then adding steps sequentially; however, training begins with the last step in the behavior chain. For example, the last step (ie, Step 15) for handwashing in **Table 1** is to dry hands with a towel. The actions required to correctly engage in this step would be taught although the child's hands would be dry already and the towel placed in his hands. Initially, the child needs to complete only the final step before accessing a reinforcer. Once the child consistently completes the last step independently, the therapist adds the penultimate step in the sequence. That is, the child would be required to grab the towel (Step 14) and dry hands with the towel (Step 15) to receive a reinforcer. Once Steps 14 and 15 are completed independently by the child, Step 13 is added. This sequence continues until all steps from beginning to end are completed independently by the child.

For both forward and backward chaining, the child is not required to complete any steps that are not currently the target of training. For example, in backward chaining, the child is not required to grab the towel if she or he is only acquiring the step of drying his or her hands with the towel. Generally, there are 3 options for the nontarget steps in a chain: (1) the child could be physically guided through the untrained steps (if necessary for the task), (2) someone else (eg, a teacher), could complete the steps for the child (this may not be possible for all tasks), or (3) the untrained steps are omitted altogether (eg, if unnecessary to complete subsequent steps).

In comparison, *total-task presentation*, a third approach to teaching a behavior chain, requires the child to complete every step of the entire behavior chain each time she or he practices the skill. The behavior chain is always taught in its correct order (ie, starts at Step 1), and the child is typically allowed an opportunity to try to complete each step independently (ie, Steps 1 through 15 in **Table 1**) before an increasing level of prompts is delivered (eg, the correct response is modeled, then partially guided, then fully guided) until the step is completed. All 3 of the methods described here can be effective in teaching behavior chains, but there may be differences in efficiency. Due to the completion of all steps in the sequence during every practice opportunity, total-task presentation can be less efficient (eg, more time consuming) than forward and backward chaining. In contrast, both forward chaining and backward chaining have been shown to be similarly efficient.[32]

Behavior chains can be taught using an *activity schedule*, which is a series of pictures, words/sentences, or a video that shows steps in the behavior chain. An everyday example of a visual activity schedule for children is the instruction manual used to build a Lego set. These visual activity schedules show a sequence of pictures and block parts that are required to build the structure at each step. Krantz and colleagues[33] used a visual activity schedule to teach children with ASD to complete various daily living skills (eg, hanging a coat, getting a snack). The children flipped pages in a binder and each page showed a step or activity to complete. Once the child finished the step on the page, he or she turned to the next page to complete another activity, and accessed the reinforcer when the child finished all activities.

One limitation of activity schedules is that the child must have access to the materials while performing the behavior chain. For some activities (eg, showering, riding a bike from one location to the next), it may be difficult to arrange an activity schedule that does not get damaged or interfere with the behavior chain; however, integrating activity schedules with technology could offer some solutions. In the United States, roughly 80% of adults own a smartphone,[34] which could provide a portable and socially valid device for activity schedules at home and in the community. An activity schedule on a smartphone or tablet may include video models and video, picture, or audio prompts.[35] For example, when teaching showering, a parent may make use of timed audio scripts or auto-advancing pictures on a tablet to make the prompts available without risking water damage.

SUMMARY

Early intervention based on the principles of ABA can improve the functioning of children with ASD by addressing behavioral deficits and excesses. Early social skills deficits, such as joint attention, can be taught in early intervention that emphasizes motivating situations and the delivery of social interactions for targeted behavior. Deficits in social communication can be resolved by using ABA language interventions that establish early verbal operants, such as echoics, mands, and tacts, and increases the complexity and social aspects of language by teaching simple and complex intraverbals. Other behavioral deficits, such as independent living skills, are also addressed through behavioral interventions such as chaining and activity schedules.

DISCLOSURE

The authors have nothing to disclose.

REFERENCES

1. American Psychiatric Association. Diagnostic and statistical manual of mental disorders (DSM-5®). Washington, DC: American Psychiatric Pub; 2013.
2. Happé F, Ronald A, Plomin R. Time to give up on a single explanation for autism. Nat Neurosci 2006;9(10):1218–20.
3. Baio J. Prevalence of autism spectrum disorder among children aged 8 years — autism and developmental disabilities monitoring network, 11 sites, United States, 2014. MMWR Surveill Summ 2018;67:1–23.
4. Center for Disease Control and Prevention. Data and statistics on autism spectrum disorder | CDC. Centers for Disease Control and Prevention Website. 2019. Available at: https://www.cdc.gov/ncbddd/autism/data.html. Accessed June 24, 2019.
5. Neimy H, Pelaez M, Carrow J, et al. Infants at risk of autism and developmental disorders: establishing early social skills. Behav Dev Bull 2017;22(1):6–22.
6. Ozonoff S, Iosif A, Baguio F, et al. A prospective study of the emergence of early behavioral signs of autism. J Am Acad Child Adolesc Psychiatry 2010;49(3): 256–66.
7. Zwaigenbaum L, Bryson S, Rogers T, et al. Behavioral manifestations of autism in the first year of life. Int J Dev Neurosci 2005;23(2):143–52.
8. Hansen SG, Carnett A, Tullis CA. Defining early social communication skills: a systematic review and analysis. Adv Neurodev Disord 2018;2(1):116–28.
9. Flynn L, Healy O. A review of treatments for deficits in social skills and self-help skills in autism spectrum disorder. Res Autism Spectr Disord 2012;6(1):431–41.
10. Mayo J, Chlebowski C, Fein DA, et al. Age of first words predicts cognitive ability and adaptive skills in children with ASD. J Autism Dev Disord 2013;43(2):253–64.
11. Toth K, Munson J, Meltzoff A N, et al. Early predictors of communication development in young children with autism spectrum disorder: joint attention, imitation, and toy play. J Autism Dev Disord 2006;36(8):993–1005.
12. Ayres KM, Mechling L, Sansosti FJ. The use of mobile technologies to assist with life skills/independence of students with moderate/severe intellectual disability and/or autism spectrum disorders: considerations for the future of school psychology. Psychol Sch 2013;50(3):259–71.
13. Hill AP, Zuckerman KE, Hagen AD, et al. Aggressive behavior problems in children with autism spectrum disorders: prevalence and correlates in a large clinical sample. Res Autism Spectr Disord 2014;8(9):1121–33.
14. Jang J, Dixon DR, Tarbox J, et al. Symptom severity and challenging behavior in children with ASD. Res Autism Spectr Disord 2011;5(3):1028–32.
15. Matson JL, Wilkins J, Macken J. The relationship of challenging behaviors to severity and symptoms of autism spectrum disorders. J Ment Health Res Intellect Disabl 2009;2(1):29–44.
16. Farmer CA, Aman MG. Aggressive behavior in a sample of children with autism spectrum disorders. Res Autism Spectr Disord 2011;5(1):317–23.
17. Smith T, Iadarola S. Evidence base update for autism spectrum disorder. J Clin Child Adolesc Psychol 2015;44(6):897–922.
18. Autism Speaks. State regulated health benefit plans. Autism Speaks Website. 2019. Available at: https://www.autismspeaks.org/state-regulated-health-benefit-plans. Accessed July 19, 2019.
19. National Autism Center. Findings and conclusions: national standards project, phase 2. Randolph (MA): National Autism Center; 2015.

20. Adamson LB, Bakeman R. Mothers' communicative acts: changes during infancy. Infant Behav Dev 1984;7(4):467–78.
21. Dube WV, Macdonald RPF, Mansfield RC, et al. Toward a behavioral analysis of joint attention. Behav Analyst 2004;27(2):197–207.
22. Carpenter M, Nagell K, Tomasello M, et al. Social cognition, joint attention, and communicative competence from 9 to 15 months of age. Monogr Soc Res Child Dev 1998;63(4). i-174.
23. Mundy P, Sigman M, Kasari C. Joint attention, developmental level, and symptom presentation in autism. Dev Psychopathol 1994;6(3):389–401.
24. Jones EA, Carr EG. Joint attention in children with autism. Focus Autism Other Dev Disabl 2004;19(1):13–26.
25. Isaksen J, Holth P. An operant approach to teaching joint attention skills to children with autism. Behav Interv 2009;24(4):215–36.
26. Taylor BA, Hoch H. Teaching children with autism to respond to and initiate bids for joint attention. J Appl Behav Anal 2008;41(3):377–91.
27. Skinner BF. Verbal behavior. Englewood Cliffs (NJ): Prentice-Hall Inc.; 1957. p. 478.
28. Sundberg ML, Michael J. The benefits of Skinner's analysis of verbal behavior for children with autism. Behav Modif 2001;25(5):698–724.
29. Sundberg ML, Sundberg CA. Intraverbal behavior and verbal conditional discriminations in typically developing children and children with autism. Anal Verbal Behav 2011;27(1):23–44.
30. Williams G, Oliver JM, Allard A, et al. Autism and associated medical and familial factors: a case control study. J Dev Phys Disabl 2003;15(4):335–49.
31. Sullivan PM, Knutson JF. Maltreatment and disabilities: a population-based epidemiological study. Child Abuse Negl 2000;24(10):1257–73.
32. Spooner F, Spooner D. A review of chaining techniques: implications for future research and practice. Educ Train Ment Retard 1984.
33. Krantz PJ, MacDuff MT, McClannahan LE. Programming participation in family activities for children with autism: parents' use of photographic activity schedules. J Appl Behav Anal 1993;26(1):137–8.
34. Pew Research Center. Demographics of mobile device ownership and adoption in the United States | Pew Research Center. 2019. Available at: https://www.pewinternet.org/fact-sheet/mobile/. Accessed July 12, 2019.
35. Goldsmith TR, LeBlanc LA. Use of technology in interventions for children with autism. J Early Intensive Behav Interv 2004;1(2):166–78.

20.

Behavioral Approaches to Weight Management for Health and Wellness

Matthew P. Normand, PhD*, Joshua Logan Gibson, BS

KEYWORDS

- Applied behavior analysis • Fitness • Health • Obesity • Wellness

KEY POINTS

- Obesity can be construed as a behavior problem insofar as it is the result of energy intake in excess of energy expenditure.
- A primary determinant of energy intake is diet and a primary determinant of energy expenditure is physical activity.
- To lose weight, you need to decrease calorie consumption, increase calorie expenditure, or both. You decrease calorie consumption by eating less and you can increase calorie expenditure by moving more.
- Behavioral interventions to increase and decrease target behaviors are relevant to the problem of obesity.
- Most behavioral interventions for obesity have involved some combination of goal setting, self-monitoring, feedback, and incentives and have produced modest short-term changes in weight, but long-term weight loss or maintenance has not been consistently demonstrated.

Obesity has become a worldwide public health crisis associated with serious health problems.[1] Obesity rates have tripled worldwide since 1975, with almost 40% of adults classified as overweight and approximately 13% as obese.[2] In the United States, recent estimates indicate that 40% of adults and 18.5% of children and adolescents are obese, and the obesity rate is more than double what it was in 1980.[3–5] If the trend continues, it is quite possible that more than one-half of the US population will be obese by 2030.[3] These numbers translate into some staggering costs to individuals and to society; approximately $147 billion is spent on obesity-related problems and those costs could soon top $956 billion.[3,6,7]

Being obese is associated with serious health problems such as coronary heart disease, hypertension, stroke, diabetes, and cancer.[8,9] For adults, being obese increases

Department of Psychology, University of the Pacific, Stockton, CA 95211, USA
* Corresponding author.
E-mail address: mnormand@pacific.edu

Pediatr Clin N Am 67 (2020) 537–546
https://doi.org/10.1016/j.pcl.2020.02.008
0031-3955/20/© 2020 Elsevier Inc. All rights reserved.

the risk of illness and death associated with those maladies, sometimes consider-ably.[10,11] For children, the associations between obesity and such maladies are less clear than they are for adults. However, young adults are increasingly being diagnosed with type 2 diabetes and the cancers most associated with obesity.[12,13] Moreover, obese adolescents often become obese adults, who then are likely to suffer from 1 or more associated health problems.[14]

OBESITY AS A BEHAVIOR PROBLEM

Obesity is a straightforward problem: energy intake in excess of energy expenditure. And energy intake and energy expenditure are, by and large, behavior problems, because you gain weight as a result of consuming more calories than you burn.[15] Although genetics undoubtedly influence weight, the rapid increase in obesity rates over the past few decades occurred far too quickly for genes to play any pivotal role.[15,16] Instead, environmental changes such as the increased availability of food, especially high-calorie foods, have interacted with our evolutionary histories that, for example, make us especially sensitive to food as a reinforcer; factors that have com-bined to produce the current epidemic.[15–18] The exceptions to this are few and ac-count for relatively little of the variance in healthy weights in the average population, or for the dramatic increase in obesity rates over the past few decades.[15,16,19,20] More-over, even the exceptions still fit into the calorie equation. Weight remains a function of calories consumed and calories burned, and this calorie equation must be managed to prevent obesity.

A FUNCTIONAL ANALYSIS OF OBESITY-RELATED BEHAVIOR

As with other behavior problems, eating too much or moving too little can result from a skills deficit, countertherapeutic motivating conditions, an obesogenic environment, or some combination thereof. The seminal paper, "The control of eating," by Ferster, Nurnberger, and Levitt[21] marked the formal introduction of a behavioral interpretation of one key component of overweight and obesity, overeating, and lead to the first sys-tematic behavioral intervention for weight loss, reported by Stuart.[22,23] Stuart succinc-tly described the basic approach, as follows:

> The first step in self-control is a precise analysis of the response to be controlled and its antecedent and consequent conditions. An analysis of overeating would natu-rally include a precise description of the topography of the response, the condi-tions under which it occurs, and its consequences. The second step is the identification of behavior which facilitates eating a proper amount of food (including behavior which interferes with overeating). The third step is the identi-fication of positive or negative reinforcers which control these behavior patterns. . . . The fourth step requires the application of the reinforcement to alter the prob-ability of the preselected response…The outcome of self-control can be termed "contingency management" and is designed to increase the frequency of desired overt or covert responses while decreasing the frequency of undesired re-sponses. (p. 357)

From a behavioral economics standpoint, eating too much and exercising too little make some sense.[24] Generally speaking, the reinforcers for healthy behavior might not be as powerful as those for unhealthy behavior, with the result being that we engage in less of the former and more of the latter. The immediate consequences of eating are powerful reinforcers related to satiety and the sensory stimuli associated with food, whereas the unwanted consequences of eating, such as weight gain, are not immediately forthcoming. The immediate consequences of exercise, such as sweating and muscle pain, can be punishing, whereas the desired consequences of exercise, such as weight loss and muscularity, are delayed and probabilistic. Thus, the natural reinforcement contingencies tend to favor unhealthy behavior for many individuals.

In light of this, a focus of the Ferster, Nurnberger, and Levitt method was to establish strong self-stated rules describing the harms resulting from poor diet to establish such rules as, among other things, a motivating statement that would decrease the value of food as a reinforcer.[21] That is, Ferster and colleagues[21] recognized that being able to describe what you should do is not the same as doing it. They also recognized that the problem is not really that we devalue delayed consequences,[25] it is that there are only immediate consequences to choose. In the case of overeating, our behavior might be controlled by the presence of food to be eaten or by things we say about eating that food, such as descriptions of the negative long-term consequences of doing so. Importantly, the long-term consequences themselves cannot control behavior because they do not yet exist; indeed, they might never come to pass. Instead, Ferster and colleagues focused on making the competing self-stated rules about healthy eating a stronger controlling variable to compete with the presence of food.[a]

Another strategy to encourage healthy behavior is to alter the environment such that discriminative stimuli related to unhealthy behavior are absent, or at least less conspicuous. So-called situational engineering includes strategies such as removing unhealthy food from the house and keeping only healthy food in the cupboards, which might lead to healthier eating by increasing the number of discriminative stimuli relevant to eating healthy food and decrease those relevant to eating unhealthy food.[22,26] However, a thorny problem with reducing eating and maintaining that reduction in this way is that, unlike many other behavior problems (eg, smoking), we have to keep eating at some level. This circumstance means that we continue to contact the reinforcers for eating and the discriminative stimuli associated with those reinforcers. We cannot simply eliminate them or provide them contingent on other, healthier behavior. Still, doing things such as packing a bag with exercise clothes and keeping the bag in the car can make it more likely that you will drive to the gym after work.[22,26]

Situational engineering also increases the response effort required for unhealthy behavior and decreases the effort required for healthy behavior. Ferster, Nurnberger, and Levitt,[21] for example, astutely noted that eating is actually a behavior chain rather than a discrete behavior. Eating involves sequences of behavior that end in chewing and swallowing food. Those sequences begin some distance away from the ultimate reinforcers and involve behaviors such as preparing the food, serving the food, picking up utensils, and so forth. Recognition of this process suggests that one could arrange events that interrupt those chains or that make those chains longer and, thus, more difficult and potentially less reinforcing because the ratio of responses to reinforcement is increased. If one were to have to cut apples, measure flour, roll dough, mix ingredients and wait for it to bake, an apple pie might be kept for special occasions, rather than a nightly dessert. Many of the strategies subsumed under situational engineering alter the sequences of behavior that end with eating or physical activity. With respect to eating, strategies such as keeping very little food in the house and keeping only food that needs to be prepared means that you will have to go buy food and engage in the steps necessary to prepare it before you eat. In this way, unhealthy

---

[a] This element of the analysis by Ferster and colleagues is not a common feature of the intervention research that followed.

activities like snacking on unhealthy food change from effortless to effortful. Alternatively, joining a gym that is on the way to work or very near your house and keeping a bag of workout clothes packed and in your car make it easier to go to the gym by decreasing the number of steps in the relevant behavior chain.

BEHAVIORAL APPROACHES TO WEIGHT MANAGEMENT

The first reports of behavioral research using weight as the primary-dependent variable were published before the so-called obesity epidemic emerged.[22,27,28] This prescient work incorporated established behavior-change techniques to promote weight loss and, as mentioned elsewhere in this article, the Ferster, Nurnberger, Levitt[21] analysis proved seminal. Shortly thereafter, Stuart[22] published the first clinical investigation of behavioral intervention to reduce overeating. That intervention was based explicitly on Ferster and colleagues's[23,29] analysis and serves as the basis for all behavioral interventions that have followed, although a number of refinements have been made over the years.

Stuart worked individually with 8 patients over the course of almost 2 years, with initial contacts occurring multiple times per week, then less often as treatment progressed.[22] The patients were taught basic principles of behavior and how to use them to change behavior, how to record the food the they ate and record their weight, and how to use specific behavior change strategies, such as situational engineering. All patients lost weight and maintained that weight loss over the course of 52 weeks.[22] Stuart, like Ferster and colleagues,[21] emphasized changing current circumstances related to overeating, specifically, and did not emphasize physical activity. Stuart also noted that his treatment differed somewhat from that described by Ferster and colleagues in several ways, including that individual rather than group therapy was arranged and teaching participants to describe the aversive consequences of obesity was not a focal point.

With Stuart, the ball was rolling and it has not slowed over the years.[23,29] One important development, however, is that the earliest behavioral interventions for obesity focused on eating as the crucial behavior and largely ignored physical activity, whereas current interventions target both eating and activity. There is debate about the extent to which exercise alone produces significant weight loss, but research does show that physical activity is important for both initial and, especially, prolonged weight loss.[30-34] And physical activity has health benefits even independent of weight loss.[35-39] Today, effective interventions involve treatment packages that target diet, exercise, and lifestyle physical activity.[40-42] More specifically, there is an increased emphasis on intensive lifestyle interventions (ILIs) that prioritize more global, and sometimes smaller, changes in diet and physical activity that are to be maintained indefinitely, rather than on acute shorter term changes in diet and exercise.[29,43-45]

Shorter term diet and exercise regimens, rather than general lifestyle changes, seem to be somewhat less effective,[46,47] perhaps in part because they require the overweight person to refrain from doing things that most others do (eg, eating dessert) or to do things that most others do not (eg, exercise daily). Also, with respect to diet, arranging food deprivation or restricted access to preferred foods might actually increase the motivation to eat, or to eat certain foods, and lead to an increased probability of unhealthy eating.[21] Smaller changes in diet that include opportunities to sometimes eat preferred unhealthy foods are thus worth considering, although this matter ultimately is empirical and to be settled via experimental research. Importantly, overall calorie reduction seems to be the operative variable; research suggests that diet composition in terms of macronutrients (fats, proteins, and carbohydrates) does not contribute to weight loss when total calories are held constant.[43] Therefore, consuming moderate amounts of preferred food does not seem to be contraindicated. Somewhat smaller lifestyle changes might also have the benefit of increasing adherence to intervention procedures, which, not surprisingly, is associated with increased weight loss.[29]

KEY FEATURES OF BEHAVIORAL INTERVENTIONS

The most evidence-based behavioral interventions to promote weight loss all include a combination of task clarification, goal setting, self-monitoring, and feedback.[23,29,44] Some interventions also include tangible incentives that are delivered for evidence of meeting specific behavioral goals.[48] In a standard behavioral intervention, the importance of maintaining a healthy weight is explained, usually with instructions for how to do so. Clear and manageable goals for weight loss are established, and clear consequences for meeting or not meeting these goals are arranged. Historically, behavior therapy interventions were delivered on an individual basis, but many programs now deliver the interventions in group formats with outcomes similar to those delivered individually.[29,49] The more successful interventions continue over multiple months or years, with success rates positively associated with intervention length, at least to some extent.[23,29,43,44,50] Some recent research suggests that telehealth delivery models, such as telephone or Internet-delivered programs, produce somewhat less weight loss than in-person programs, but not substantially so.[43,50] Any losses in effectiveness might be offset by increased availability and decreased costs associated with telehealth models, making them promising approaches to intervention delivery.[44]

In terms of the specific procedures involved, task clarification can include explanations of how eating and physical activity are related to health and wellness and clarify the characteristics of healthy eating and healthy activity. Once the relevant behavioral goals are established, objectives can be set by specifying the type and amount of behavior, such as eating vegetables or walking around the neighborhood, that is to occur, and the times at which, and the circumstances in which, it should occur. Ideally, some form of self-monitoring will be arranged, such as the use of food diaries for eating, and activity monitors (eg, pedometers[51]) for physical activity.[49] Such measures provide immediate performance feedback to the individual, and self-monitoring has proven to be the most common and potentially important component of behavioral interventions for weight loss.[44] Self-monitoring (eg, using wearable activity monitors) can be supplemented by interventionist-delivered feedback consisting of descriptions of behavior change in the context of health, suggestions for further changes, praise for changes already made, and so on. The measures recorded (eg, in food diaries or via activity monitors) also can be summarized, such as on a graph, and displayed, publicly or privately.

If necessary, incentives such as money, gift cards, and the like can be arranged for meeting specified performance goals.[48] Alternatively, money or goods can be deposited up front and earned back or forfeited depending on performance.[27,28] Indeed, such incentive-based contingency management interventions have proved to be especially effective ways to promote weight loss.[48,52] For example, in one of the earliest behavioral interventions to promote weight loss, Mann[28] used contingency contracts that required participants to deposit valuable personal property that could be earned back only by meeting weight - loss goals. Missing a weight loss goal resulted in 1 or more items being forfeited. Overall, participants lost weight during the contingency contract intervention and gained weight during baseline conditions.

A bit later, Aragona and colleagues[27] used similar contingency contracts with parents of overweight children to promote weight loss in those children. The parents lost some of the money they deposited each time they failed to attend the weekly meetings, submit a weekly homework assignment, or when their child did not meet a weight goal. All children in the study lost weight over the course of the intervention. More recent research has clearly established incentive-based behavioral interventions as effective ways to promote weight loss.[48]

OVERVIEW OF CONTEMPORARY BEHAVIORAL INTERVENTION MODELS

Several large-scale behavioral intervention programs that incorporate the general features described above have been developed and formally evaluated over the past 2 decades. For example, the Diabetes Prevention Program was a large-scale, randomized clinical trial in which prediabetic adults were enrolled in 1 of 3 groups: ILI, metformin (a drug used to lower blood sugar), or placebo.[53] The ILI group received individually tailored behavioral skills training on diet and exercise, and the other 2 groups received brief standard diabetes education and either metformin or a placebo. Researchers primarily used fasting plasma glucose levels to assess the intervention; however, body weight was also measured, along with self-reports of leisure physical activity. Although the incidence of diabetes was 38% lower in the metformin group than in the placebo group, the reduced incidence of disease was even greater (58%) in the ILI group. Data collected on secondary measures showed a larger initial reduction in body weight in the ILI group compared with metformin and placebo, at an average of 5.6, 2.1, and 0.1 kg., respectively. Participants in the ILI group reported engaging in leisure physical activity up to 4 times as much as participants in the other groups.

Similarly, Look AHEAD was an 8-year, intensive program consisting of one-on-one behavioral counseling sessions, group meetings, portion-controlled meal plans, meal replacements, and prescribed exercise protocols.[54–56] For those participants who did not respond to the initial treatment package, researchers implemented a specialized set of procedures that included motivational interviewing, teaching problem solving skills, and writing behavioral contracts with the participant.[54] At 1 year, body weight reductions in the ILI group averaged 7.8% compared with 0.7% in the control group, which received standard diabetes care and education. Weight loss tapered off at 4 to 8 years, but a significant difference between the ILI and control groups remained. The ILI group had improved biomarkers for glucose and blood lipids, along with lower blood pressure, less liver fat, less kidney disease, less reliance on diabetes medication, and lower health care costs.[55]

Finally, the POUNDS Lost study lasted 2 years and placed overweight adults into 1 of 4 diet groups, each assigned a diet consisting of a different macro nutrient percentage.[57] Carbohydrates ranged from 35% to 65% of the diet, and the remainder of calories consumed were classified as low fat/average protein, low fat/high protein, high fat/average protein, or high fat/high protein. The macronutrient profiles varied, but each diet represented a deficit of 750 kcals, was low in cholesterol, low in saturated fat, and high in dietary fiber. All groups received group counseling sessions involving behavioral counseling methods on a weekly basis during the first 6 months, and biweekly sessions for the remainder of the intervention. Additionally, individual counseling sessions were held every 2 months for the duration of the intervention. Participants recorded their food and beverage intake and used an online self-monitoring program that provided feedback about their daily food intake in relation to their dietary goals. At the conclusion of the study, there were no significant differences among groups in terms of weight loss; all 4 diets were associated with an 8% weight loss after 1 year and an additional 6% weight loss after 2 years. Additionally, indicators of cardiovascular health improved to a similar degree across all groups.

SUMMARY

The preponderance of empirical evidence shows that behavioral interventions focused on promoting healthy eating and physical activity promote weight loss, although the longer term effects are less clear.[23,29,44,50] Not surprisingly, the success of any behavioral intervention for weight loss, including those described in this article, seems to be strongly related to treatment adherence.[29] Therefore, future research should perhaps focus less on refining our current intervention efforts and more on increasing intervention adherence. At the end of the day, however, an ounce of prevention is worth a pound of cure. This tenet seems especially true for overweight and obesity because maintaining weight loss seems to be such an elusive intervention goal. Unfortunately, the evidence supporting current behavioral prevention programs is not strong and prevention efforts are likely to require more nuanced individual and group interventions, in concert with policy-level interventions.[58,59] Much more work is needed in this regard.

As B. F. Skinner noted, we are, in a sense, hostages to our genetic history.[17,60] In a relatively short period of time, we have created an obesogenic environment that supersedes our evolutionary history. More so than at any time in our evolutionary past, it is easy to eat too much and move too little; thus, many of us gain too much weight. The problem is a behavior problem and the solution is behavior change: eat less and move more. Applied behavior analysis, including behavior therapy, has produced a range of methods and technologies well-suited to address a myriad of behavior problems, including overeating and physical inactivity.[61–63] The earliest behavioral attempts to understand and treat overweight and obesity proved fruitful, spawning decades of intervention research that has proved promising, if not perfect.[21,22]

DISCLOSURE

The authors have nothing to disclose.

REFERENCES

1. Kopelman PG. Obesity as a medical problem. Nature 2000;404(6778):635.
2. World Health Organization. Obesity and overweight. 2018. Available at: https://www.who.int/news-room/fact-sheets/detail/obesity-and-overweight. Accessed July 31, 2019.
3. Finkelstein EA, Khavjou OA, Thompson H, et al. Obesity and severe obesity forecasts through 2030. Am J Prev Med 2012;42(6):563–70.
4. Fryar CD, Kruszan-Moran D, Gu Q, et al. Mean body weight, weight, waist circumference, and body mass index among adults: United States, 1999–2000 through 2015–2016. Hyattsville (MD): National Center for Health Statistics.; 2018.
5. Hales CM, Carroll MD, Fryar CD, et al. Prevalence of obesity among adults and youth: United States, 2015-2016. Hyattsville (MD): National Center for Health Statistics; 2017.
6. Wang Y, Beydoun MA, Liang L, et al. Will all Americans become overweight or obese? Estimating the progression and cost of the US obesity epidemic. Obesity (Silver Spring) 2008;16(10):2323–30.

7. Finkelstein EA, Trogdon JG, Cohen JW, et al. Annual medical spending attributable to obesity: payer-and service-specific estimates. Health Aff 2009;28(5): w822–31.
8. Mokdad AH, Ford ES, Bowman BA, et al. Prevalence of obesity, diabetes, and obesity-related health risk factors, 2001. JAMA 2003;289(1):76–9.
9. Must A, Spadano J, Coakley EH, et al. The disease burden associated with overweight and obesity. JAMA 1999;282(16):1523–9.
10. Di Angelantonio E, Bhupathiraju SN, Wormser D, et al. Body-mass index and all-cause mortality: individual-participant-data meta-analysis of 239 prospective studies in four continents. Lancet 2016;388(10046):776–86.
11. American College of Cardiology/American Heart Association Task Force on Practice Guidelines. Expert panel report: guidelines (2013) for the management of overweight and obesity in adults. Obesity 2014;22:S41.
12. Sung H, Siegel RL, Rosenberg PS, et al. Emerging cancer trends among young adults in the USA: analysis of a population-based cancer registry. Lancet Public Health 2019;4(3):e137–47.
13. Mayers-Davis EJ, Lawrence JM, Dabelea D, et al. Incidence trends of type 1 and type 2 diabetes among youths, 2002–2012. N Engl J Med 2017;376(15):1419–29.
14. Simmonds M, Llewellyn A, Owen C, et al. Predicting adult obesity from childhood obesity: a systematic review and meta-analysis. Obes Rev 2016;17(2):95–107.
15. Hill JO, Peters JC. Environmental contributions to the obesity epidemic. Science 1998;280(5368):1371–4.
16. Hill JO, Wyatt HR, Reed GW, et al. Obesity and the environment: where do we go from here? Science 2003;299(5608):853–5.
17. Skinner BF. The evolution of behavior. J Exp Anal Behav 1984;41(2):217–21.
18. French SA, Story M, Jeffery RW. Environmental influences on eating and physical activity. Annu Rev Public Health 2001;22(1):309–35.
19. Bouchard C. Defining the genetic architecture of the predisposition to obesity: a challenging but not insurmountable task. Am J Clin Nutr 2010;91(1):5–6.
20. Choquet H, Meyre D. Genetics of obesity: what have we learned? Curr Genomics 2011;12(3):169–79.
21. Ferster CB, Nurnberger JI, Levitt EB. The control of eating. 1962. Obes Res 1996; 4(4):401–10.
22. Stuart RB. Behavioral control of overeating. Behav Res Ther 1967;5(4):357–65.
23. Wilson GT. Behavioral treatment of obesity: thirty years and counting. Behav Res Ther 1994;16(1):31–75.
24. Bickel WK, Vuchinich RE. Reframing health behavior change with behavioral economics. Mahwah (NJ): Lawrence Erlbaum Associates, Inc.; 2000.
25. Epstein LH, Salvy SJ, Carr KA, et al. Food reinforcement, delay discounting and obesity. Physiol Behav 2010;100(5):438–45.
26. Loro AD Jr, Fisher EB Jr, Levenkron JC. Comparison of established and innovative weight-reduction treatment procedures. J Appl Behav Anal 1979;12:141–55.
27. Aragona J, Cassady J, Drabman RS. Treating overweight children through parental training and contingency contracting. J Appl Behav Anal 1975;8:269–78.
28. Mann RA. The behavior-therapeutic use of contingency contracting to control an adult behavior problem: weight control. J Appl Behav Anal 1972;5:99–109.
29. Williamson DA. Fifty years of behavioral/lifestyle interventions for overweight and obesity: where have we been and where are we going? Obesity 2017;25(11): 1867–75.
30. Hill JO, Wyatt HR. Role of physical activity in preventing and treating obesity. J Appl Physiol 2005;99(2):765–70.

31. Jeffery RW, Wing RR, Sherwood NE, et al. Physical activity and weight loss: does prescribing higher physical activity goals improve outcome? Am J Clin Nutr 2003; 78(4):684–9.

32. Catenacci VA, Wyatt HR. The role of physical activity in producing and maintaining weight loss. Nat Rev Endocrinol 2007;3(7):518.

33. Wu T, Gao X, Chen M, et al. Long term effectiveness of diet plus exercise interventions vs. diet only interventions for weight loss: a meta analysis. Obes Rev 2009;10(3):313–23.

34. Curioni C, Lourenco P. Long-term weight loss after diet and exercise: a systematic review. Int J Obes 2005;29(10):1168–74.

35. Reiner M, Niermann C, Jekauc D, et al. Long-term health benefits of physical activity–a systematic review of longitudinal studies. BMC Public Health 2013; 13:813.

36. Väistö J, Eloranta A-M, Viitasalo A, et al. Physical activity and sedentary behaviour in relation to cardiometabolic risk in children: cross-sectional findings from the Physical Activity and Nutrition in Children (PANIC) Study. Int J Behav Nutr Phys Act 2014;11:55.

37. Warburton DE, Nicol CW, Bredin SS. Health benefits of physical activity: the evidence. Can Med Assoc J 2006;174(6):801–9.

38. World Health Organization. Physical activity. World Health Organization. 2018. Available at: http://www.who.int/news-room/fact-sheets/detail/physical-activity. Accessed July 18, 2018.

39. Centers for Disease Control and Prevention. Physical activity and health. Centers for Disease Control and Prevention. 2018. Available at: https://www.cdc.gov/physicalactivity/basics/pa-health/index.htm. Accessed July 18, 2018.

40. Epstein LH, Valoski A, Wing RR, et al. Ten-year outcomes of behavioral family-based treatment for childhood obesity. Health Psychol 1994;13(5):373.

41. Epstein LH, Paluch RA, Roemmich JN, et al. Family-based obesity treatment, then and now: twenty-five years of pediatric obesity treatment. Health Psychol 2007;26(4):381–91.

42. Jakicic JM, Clark K, Coleman E, et al. Appropriate intervention strategies for weight loss and prevention of weight regain for adults. Med Sci Sports Exerc 2001;33(12):2145–56.

43. Wadden TA, Butryn ML, Wilson C. Lifestyle modification for the management of obesity. Gastroenterology 2007;132(6):2226–38.

44. Wadden TA, Webb VL, Moran CH, et al. Lifestyle modification for obesity: new developments in diet, physical activity, and behavior therapy. Circulation 2012; 125(9):1157–70.

45. Webb VL, Wadden TA. Intensive lifestyle intervention for obesity: principles, practices, and results. Gastroenterology 2017;152(7):1752–64.

46. Pagoto SL, Appelhans BM. A call for an end to the diet debates. JAMA 2013; 310(7):687–8.

47. Ho M, Garnett SP, Baur L, et al. Effectiveness of lifestyle interventions in child obesity: systematic review with meta-analysis. Pediatrics 2012;130(6):e1647–71.

48. Jeffery RW. Financial incentives and weight control. Prev Med 2012;55(Suppl): S61–7.

49. Appel LJ, Clark JM, Yeh H-C, et al. Comparative effectiveness of weight-loss interventions in clinical practice. N Engl J Med 2011;365(21):1959–68.

50. Butryn ML, Webb V, Wadden TA. Behavioral treatment of obesity. Psychiatr Clin North Am 2011;34(4):841–59.

51. Normand MP. Increasing physical activity through self-monitoring, goal setting, and feedback. Behav Interv 2008;23(4):227–36.
52. Petry NM, Barry D, Pescatello L, et al. A low-cost reinforcement procedure improves short-term weight loss outcomes. Am J Med 2011;124(11):1082–5.
53. Knowler WC, Barrett-Connor E, Fowler SE, et al. Reduction in the incidence of type 2 diabetes with lifestyle intervention or metformin. N Engl J Med 2002; 346(6):393–403.
54. The Look AHEAD Research Group. The look AHEAD study: a description of the lifestyle intervention and the evidence supporting it. Obesity 2006;14(5):737–52.
55. The Look AHEAD Research Group. Eight year weight losses with an intensive lifestyle intervention: the look AHEAD study. Obesity 2014;22(1):5–13.
56. The Look AHEAD Research Group. Look AHEAD (Action for Health in Diabetes): design and methods for a clinical trial of weight loss for the prevention of cardiovascular disease in type 2 diabetes. Control Clin Trials 2003;24(5):610–28.
57. Sacks FM, Bray GA, Carey VJ, et al. Comparison of weight-loss diets with different compositions of fat, protein, and carbohydrates. N Engl J Med 2009; 360(9):859–73.
58. Wadden TA, Brownell KD, Foster GD. Obesity: responding to the global epidemic. J Consult Clin Psychol 2002;70(3):510.
59. Kamath CC, Vickers KS, Ehrlich A, et al. Behavioral interventions to prevent childhood obesity: a systematic review and metaanalyses of randomized trials. J Clin Endocrinol Metab 2008;93(12):4606–15.
60. Chance P. Learning and behavior. 7th edition. Belmont (CA): Wadsworth; 2014.
61. Fisher WW, Piazza CC, Roane HS. Handbook of applied behavior analysis. New York: Guilford Press; 2011.
62. Roane HS, Ringdahl JE, Falcomata TS. Clinical and organizational applications of applied behavior analysis. San Diego (CA): Elsevier Academic Press; 2015.
63. Madden GJ, Dube WV, Hackenberg TD, et al. APA handbook of behavior analysis: translating principles into practice, vol. 2. Washington, DC: American Psychological Association; 2013.

Pediatric Prevention
Tic Disorders

Jordan T. Stiede, BA[a], Douglas W. Woods, PhD[b],*

KEYWORDS

• Tourette disorder • Tics • Children • Behavior therapy • CBIT

KEY POINTS

- It is not clear whether the development of tics can be prevented, but individuals with tics may be able to use various strategies to prevent the worsening of tics.
- Teaching families to shift attention to behaviors that reduce tics instead of attending to tics is an important part of decreasing tic severity.
- Various medications can serve as treatment options to reduce tic severity.
- Behavioral treatment is the gold standard psychotherapy intervention for tic disorders, with multiple studies demonstrating its efficacy and few side effects.
- CBIT is the most well-supported nonpharmacological treatment for children with tics.

INTRODUCTION

Tourette disorder (TD) is a childhood-onset neurologic condition, which involves the performance of sudden, repetitive, nonrhythmic motor movements and vocalizations that persist for at least 1 year.[1] The disorder is more prevalent in males, and cross-cultural studies suggest that it occurs in about 0.5% to 1% of youth.[2–5] The condition is believed to result from failed inhibition within cortico-striatal-thalamo-cortical circuits, because abnormally active striatal neurons in the basal ganglia lead to the release of unwanted motor movements and vocalizations.[6]

Although tic disorders have a neurologic basis, studies demonstrate that the environmental context plays a significant role in tic expression. Contextual factors, such as particular settings, participating in activities, reactions of other people to tics, and emotions have all been found to impact tic severity.[7] These variables interact with biological processes to help explain the variability in tics. Typical tic onset occurs between the ages 5 and 7 years, and tics tend to increase in frequency and intensity until children are approximately 10 to 11 years.[2,8–10] Tics are categorized into simple and complex, motor and vocal movements. Most tics are simple movements or

[a] Psychology Department, Marquette University, Cramer Hall, 307, PO Box 1881, Milwaukee, WI 53201-1881, USA; [b] Marquette University, Holthusen Hall, 305, PO Box 1881, Milwaukee, WI 5320-1881, USA
* Corresponding author.
E-mail address: douglas.woods@marquette.edu

Pediatr Clin N Am 67 (2020) 547–557
https://doi.org/10.1016/j.pcl.2020.02.009
0031-3955/20/© 2020 Elsevier Inc. All rights reserved.

vocalizations, such as eye blinks, head jerks, throat clears, or grunts; however, other tics involve coordinated actions by multiple muscle groups. Examples of complex tics can include fixed sequences of simple tics, touching and tapping, and various vocalizations.

Premonitory urges, uncomfortable physical sensations, such as an itch or a burn, often precede tics.[11] Such experiences are reported by over 90% of individuals with tics, and children often experience but cannot reliably report urges until approximately age 10 years.[12] Premonitory urges may occur in specific regions of the body where the tic occurs, or they may be experienced as "generalized" across the entire body. The uncomfortable sensation is usually relieved by the completion of the tic, and some individuals describe the urge to be more bothersome than the actual tic.[13]

Children and adolescents seeking treatment of TD usually have mild to moderate tic severity and impairment related to tics.[13,14] Tic severity is greatest around age 10 years, with close to 85% of individuals reporting a reduction in severity as they enter adolescence and young adulthood.[9,15] In a longitudinal study by Bloch and colleagues,[15] approximately 33% of participants were tic free by late adolescence, and less than 25% showed mild or greater tic severity according to the Yale Global Tic Severity Scale.[16] Furthermore, studies have shown that more severe tics are positively correlated with tic-related impairment in multiple settings.[17,18] Unsurprisingly, tics greater in number, frequency, intensity, complexity, and interference usually are more distressing and difficult to manage at home, in school, and in other public places.[19] Stiede and colleagues[18] also demonstrated that motor tic complexity and vocal tic number and intensity tend to contribute the most to impairment.

Although TD is defined by tics, co-occurring conditions are often present. Approximately 78% to 90% of individuals with TD experience one or more comorbidities, with attention deficit-hyperactivity disorder (ADHD) and obsessive-compulsive disorder (OCD) being the most common.[2,14,20–22] Comorbid ADHD is present in 30% to 50% of people with TD, and 10% to 50% have OCD.[20,23] Children with TD are also at a higher risk for anxiety disorders, oppositional defiant disorder, and mood disorders.[2,20] Studies have demonstrated that lower quality of life, lower self-esteem, and poorer social functioning are more common for individuals with tics plus comorbidities than individuals with only tics.[24–26]

VARIABLES AFFECTING THE EXPRESSION OF TICS

It is not clear whether the development of tics can be prevented, but individuals with tics may be able to use various strategies to prevent the worsening of tics and related psychosocial problems. Numerous studies have examined the role behavior therapy can play in tic management. The behavioral model suggests that settings (eg, school, home, friend's house), activities (eg, sports, music), the presence or absence of specific stimuli (eg, people, emotions, sensations), and reactions of other people to tics (eg, parents, peers) can all directly influence the occurrence of tics.[7] These contextual variables can be broken down into antecedent and consequence factors.

Antecedents are external or internal events that occur before tics that may change the likelihood of tic expression.[7] Settings, activities, and other people are examples of external antecedents. Studies have suggested that watching television and playing video games are associated with increases in tic expression, whereas concentrating on artistic or creative activities, such as painting, taking photographs, and playing/listening to music, are related to reductions in tics.[27–30] Internal antecedents include feelings, such as stress, boredom, anger, and frustration. Himle and colleagues[31] demonstrated that stressful situations worsened tics in 74% of children. Similarly,

Silva and colleagues[30] showed that anxiety-producing situations, such as starting a new school year, waiting for test results, and family conflict were the most common factors that increased tic severity.

Consequence variables are events that occur in reaction to tics. Studies suggest that reactions to tics can maintain or strengthen future probability of tics via positive or negative reinforcement.[7] For example, Capriotti and colleagues[32] demonstrated that social-based (eg, another kid teases child; parent gives child a hug) and escape-based (eg, child allowed to stop doing homework) consequences of tics were positively correlated with several dimensions of tic severity. Himle and colleagues[31] also showed that attention-based reactions to tics (eg, consoling, telling a child to stop ticcing) were related to increases in tic frequency. Furthermore, Watson and Sterling[33] examined the relationship between parental attention and the prevalence of a 4-year-old child's coughing tic. Results demonstrated that parental attention for the tic was associated with greater tic severity, whereas positive parental attention for the absence of the tic led to a decrease in tic expression. Combined, these studies suggest that reactions to mild tics may further exacerbate them, and actively ignoring tics may prevent the worsening of symptoms over time and lead to a less severe course.

Eaton and colleagues[34] examined the relationship between internalizing symptoms, reactions to tics, and tic severity. Results showed that children with higher levels of internalizing symptoms experienced more reactions to tics. In particular, children's total anxiety symptoms (ie, separation anxiety and social anxiety) were significantly positively correlated with consequences they received for their tics and total tic severity. Results also demonstrated that children with persistent tic disorders and increased depression received more accommodations for and reactions to displaying tics. Finally, a regression analysis indicated that total environmental consequences was a significant predictor of total tic severity. Overall, these studies suggest that teaching families to shift attention to behaviors that reduce tics instead of attending to tics is an important part of decreasing tic severity. Families that do not learn this concept run the potential risk of creating an environment that could exacerbate tics. In addition, with multiple studies demonstrating the influence of stress/anxiety on tics, the use of relaxation techniques may be beneficial.

There is also some evidence that the ability of children with recent-onset tics to suppress their tics can predict future tic severity. Kim and colleagues[35] had 45 children with recent-onset tics complete multiple tic suppression tasks in which they were asked to tic freely, to inhibit their tics, and to inhibit their tics in the presence of a reward. Researchers examined the children's tic severity at baseline and at a 12-month follow-up. Results showed that participants who showed better tic suppression in the presence of a reward exhibited reduced tic severity at the 12-month follow-up visit. These results suggest that better tic-inhibitory ability at tic onset may be associated with longer-term remission and/or reduction of tics, but future studies are needed to confirm this claim. Interestingly, simply asking a child to inhibit tics in the absence of a reward did not predict future tic outcome; therefore, the reward seems to be a key element in reducing the expression of tics.

TREATMENT OPTIONS

Because ADHD and OCD are often more impairing than tics, and these comorbidities can influence the effectiveness of behavioral treatment, such comorbid conditions should be managed before tic-specific treatment begins.[36,37] Furthermore, if children have provisional or mild tics, psychoeducation about tic disorders and the impact of the environment on tics may be enough to alleviate concerns.[38] However, if tics are associated with impairment, such as distress in school, bullying, or physical pain, then behavior therapy and pharmacotherapy are the 2 primary evidence-based interventions that should be considered.

Recently, the American Academy of Neurology (AAN) published recommendations for the assessment and treatment of tics, which were established by a multidisciplinary panel of tic experts.[39] The panel recommended that alpha-agonists should be considered in the treatment of tics, and that antipsychotic medication may be considered when the benefits of treatment outweigh the risks. Similarly, relative to other initial treatment options, such as other psychosocial/behavioral interventions and medication, the most well-supported behavioral treatment, Comprehensive Behavioral Intervention for Tics (CBIT), should be considered when treating tics.

Medication

Several medications serve as treatment options for tics. For milder tics, nonneuroleptic medications, such as clonidine and guanfacine, are the recommended option. These alpha-2 adrenergic agonists are regularly used to treat tics because they have relatively few side effects, but their effectiveness in reducing tic severity is usually modest.[40]

For more severe tics, typical (eg, haloperidol, pimozide) and atypical neuroleptics (eg, aripiprazole, risperidone) seem to be more effective than alpha-2 adrenergic agonists in reducing tic severity.[41] The efficacy of traditional neuroleptics (eg, haloperidol, pimozide, fluphenazine) has been demonstrated in multiple placebo-controlled trials.[42–44] In addition, studies suggested that pimozide may have fewer side effects than haloperidol.[45,46] Atypical neuroleptics, such as risperidone and aripiprazole have also been shown to be more effective than placebo, equally effective to pimozide and clonidine, and helpful for individuals with neuropsychiatric comorbidities.[41] Unfortunately, side effects, such as dyskinesia, acute dystonia, depression, weight gain, drowsiness, and cardiac concerns can occur.[41] Although these medications can reduce up to 70% of tics, side effects may restrict their use.[47]

Other Emerging Medical Therapies

Although not rated as having high empirical support in the AAN review, there are other emerging medical therapies with some evidence for reducing tic severity. Recent studies have shown that tetrabenazine and deutetrabenazine may improve tic severity.[48–50] Furthermore, patients with severe TD who have unsuccessfully tried medication and behavior therapy may benefit from deep brain stimulation (DBS), a treatment in which a neurostimulator sends electrical impulses into areas within the brain that have been associated with tics. Studies with adult patients have demonstrated decreases in tic severity after DBS; however, research on DBS for children is minimal.[51,52] Finally, although there is some evidence that cannabinoids can significantly reduce tics, to date there is little evidence that cannabis-based medication reduces tics in youth.[53,54]

Behavior Therapy

Behavioral treatment is considered the gold standard psychotherapy intervention for tic disorders, with multiple randomized controlled trials demonstrating its efficacy and no side effects reported.[36,38] Habit reversal training (HRT), a type of behavior therapy, has shown efficacy in multiple clinical trials and meta-analyses.[55–58] Initially, it included 14 components, but Woods and colleagues[59] suggested that awareness training, competing response training, and social support are the 3 main therapeutic skills needed for the intervention. CBIT extended HRT to include psychoeducation and functional assessment/interventions.

Currently, CBIT is the most well-supported nonpharmacological treatment for children with tics.[36,37,39,60] CBIT consists of psychoeducation, functional assessment/intervention, HRT, relaxation training, and a motivational reward program.[61] In CBIT, therapists first provide the client with psychoeducation about tic disorders to minimize blame, stigma, and negative feelings related to the client's symptoms. Next, a functional assessment is completed to assess how the environment may impact tic expression. The therapist and client discuss internal and external antecedents, such as emotions, settings, and activities that are associated with increases in tic severity. For those antecedents identified as being associated with tic exacerbation, therapists examine attention, aversive, and escape-based consequences to tics that occur within these identified antecedents.

Following the functional assessment, functional interventions are developed to manage the antecedents and consequences associated with worsening tic severity.[61] Next, the clinician implements HRT for each tic, which involves 3 elements. First, awareness training is completed to teach the client to recognize each tic and its associated premonitory urge. This step is important because if clients are not aware of their tics/urges, then it will be difficult to implement competing response exercises. After clients are aware of approximately 80% of tic occurrence, competing response training begins. Competing responses are behaviors that are physically incompatible with the target tic. Clients are instructed to use the competing response contingent on the tic or premonitory urge for 1 minute or until the urge goes away, whichever is longer. Finally, social support training is introduced to teach a social support person, in most cases a parent, how to assist the child in the implementation of the competing response. The support person's job is to praise correct implementation of the competing response and to prompt the children when they forget to do their competing response.[61]

Piacentini and colleagues[62] demonstrated that CBIT is more effective than nonspecific supportive therapy in reducing tics and tic-related impairment in children with tic disorders, with 53% of participants showing significant improvement at the end of the 8-week intervention and 87% of responders exhibiting continued benefit 6 months after treatment. Furthermore, Woods and colleagues[63] showed that CBIT does not lead to adverse effects on disruptive behavior, attention, mood, and anxiety regulation, and Rizzo and colleagues[64] suggested that behavior therapy is as effective as neuroleptic medication in treating children and adolescents with tics.

Exposure and response prevention (ERP) for tics is another behavior therapy shown to reduce tics.[65,66] In ERP, clients are asked to suppress their tics for gradually longer periods of time, with each 2-hour session consisting of exposure to sensory experiences and response prevention of tics. Unlike CBIT, all tics are targeted at once, and the therapist uses techniques, such as focusing on the urge, talking about tics, and describing situations or activities related to increases in tics, to elicit the premonitory urge. When tics occur, the therapist encourages the client to try even harder to suppress the tics, reminding them of what they would gain if they ignore the urge to tic. In a randomized controlled trial (RCT), Verdellen and colleagues[66] found no differences in posttreatment tic severity scores between participants given ERP or HRT. Pringsheim and colleagues[39] noted that if CBIT is unavailable, ERP may be an acceptable behavioral intervention.

DISSEMINATION OF BEHAVIOR THERAPY

Although CBIT is effective at reducing tic severity and is rated as highly acceptable by clients, accessibility remains a problem.[67] A survey by Woods and colleagues[68] demonstrated that most clients desire CBIT, but only approximately 6% of treatment-seeking children/families and 4% of treatment-seeking adults have received CBIT. The most common reason given for not receiving CBIT was a lack of knowledgeable and trained providers. Because CBIT's limited availability, efforts have been made to enhance its dissemination using telehealth and a self-guided Web-based treatment. Because there are few providers trained in CBIT, these adaptations could provide greater access to the intervention.

To examine the effectiveness of CBIT delivered via telehealth, Himle and colleagues[67] had 20 children with TD complete 10 weeks of CBIT delivered either face-to-face or via videoconferencing. Regardless of format, individuals demonstrated significant equivalent decreases in tic severity, which suggests that receiving telehealth CBIT is a viable option for therapy. TicHelper.com ("TicHelper") is another treatment option if CBIT providers are inaccessible. TicHelper is an online, interactive self-help program, based on CBIT, for individuals with tics from 8 years old to adolescence.[69] The program was developed using an iterative testing and feedback process involving CBIT professionals, children with persistent tics, and their parents. An RCT comparing TicHelper with an Internet-based resources condition has been completed but has not yet been published. However, the site is based on the therapist manual used in Piacentini and colleagues,[62] who showed that CBIT is more effective in reducing tics and tic-related impairment in children than supportive therapy.

In another attempt to disseminate CBIT treatment, the Tourette Association of America (TA) offers the TA-Behavior Therapy Institute, a 2-day in-person didactic and skills-based training for licensed social workers, health, or mental health practitioners.[70] After the training, each attendee can participate in 3 consultation calls with CBIT experts to discuss their training cases. An online training program, based on the CBIT manual, is also being developed to provide therapists with another opportunity to become trained in CBIT.

PREDICTORS OF TREATMENT OUTCOME

Few studies have examined moderators and predictors of response to behavior therapy for children with tic disorders. Sukhodolsky and colleagues[71] used data from 2 studies that compared CBIT with psychoeducation and supportive therapy to investigate moderators and predictors of treatment response. The combined sample consisted of 248 participants (177 male; 71 female), and selected variables included presence of baseline tic medication, tic phenomenology, age, sex, family functioning, treatment expectancy, and co-occurring ADHD, OCD, and anxiety disorders. Results demonstrated that the treatment effect of CBIT was significantly larger for participants not on tic medication compared with those on tic medication; yet, participants on tic medication still showed improvements with CBIT. The remaining variables tested did not moderate outcome.

Furthermore, Sukhodolsky and colleagues[71] suggested that co-occurring anxiety disorders, severity of premonitory urges, participant positive expectancy, and higher overall severity, as measured by the Clinical Global Impression – Severity (CGI-S), predicted tic severity outcomes regardless of treatment assignment. For example, individuals with a comorbid anxiety disorder demonstrated less tic reduction after 10 weeks of treatment. Similar results were found by Nissen and colleagues[72] who showed that high anxiety scores predicted less improvement in functional impairment after treatment. Thus, although relaxation training is an element of the behavioral program, these findings suggest that additional techniques to manage anxiety and stress may be beneficial for individuals with tics.

Premonitory urge severity was associated with lower tic reduction, suggesting that it may be more difficult for children with stronger premonitory urges to manage tics.[71] Furthermore, Sukhodolsky and colleagues[71] showed that optimism related to treatment outcome may be an important factor, as parents' and children's positive expectancy for change was associated with greater tic reduction. Similarly, Nissen and colleagues[72] demonstrated that patients who believed that it is extremely difficult to suppress tics, experienced poorer treatment outcome. Therefore, building rapport with clients to increase optimism and beginning HRT with a tic in which there is a better chance for success may be important elements for better treatment outcome. Both of these factors are emphasized in CBIT. Finally, Sukhodolsky and colleagues[71] showed that participants with higher initial tic severity demonstrated greater tic reduction over time regardless of treatment condition.

Deckersbach and colleagues[73] also examined predictors of treatment response. They used a visuospatial priming task to investigate whether pretreatment response inhibition impairment in individuals given HRT predicted reductions in tic severity. Results suggested that participants with greater deficits in response inhibition did not respond as well to HRT, suggesting that it may be harder for individuals with poor baseline response inhibition to use competing response exercises. Similarly, other studies have found that attention problems are related to poorer tic suppressibility; thus, problems with attention could predict poorer response to behavioral treatments.[74,75]

SUMMARY

Although there is no information on how to prevent the development of tics, various strategies have been shown to be effective in secondary and tertiary prevention of tics and related psychosocial problems. A behavioral model indicates that contextual variables can impact tic expression; therefore, functional assessments are used to identify antecedents and consequences related to tic exacerbation and attenuation. Functional interventions also are used to modify antecedents and consequences associated with greater tic severity. Furthermore, medication can be prescribed to reduce tic severity; however, side effects may restrict their use. Finally, in CBIT, competing responses are implemented to give individuals an exercise that they can use when they feel the urge to tic. Overall, although children may be unable to prevent the development of tics, they can still use several strategies to reduce their tic severity and impairment.

DISCLOSURE

D.W. Woods receives royalties from Oxford University Press, Springer Press, and Guilford Press. He also gives paid talks for the Tourette Association of America. J.T. Stiede has nothing to disclose.

REFERENCES

1. American Psychiatric Association. Diagnostic and statistical manual of mental disorders. 5th edirion. Washington, DC: American Psychiatric Association; 2013.
2. Freeman RD, Fast DK, Burd L, et al. An international perspective on Tourette syndrome: selected findings from 3500 individuals in 22 countries. Dev Med Child Neurol 2000;42:436–47.

3. Khalifa N, Von Knorring AL. Prevalence of tic disorders and Tourette syndrome in a Swedish school population. Dev Med Child Neurol 2003;45:315–9.

4. Knight T, Steeves T, Day L, et al. Prevalence of tic disorders: a systematic review and meta-analysis. Pediatr Neurol 2012;47:77–90.

5. Scharf JM, Miller LL, Mathews CA, et al. Prevalence of Tourette syndrome and chronic tics in the population-based Avon longitudinal study of parents and children cohort. J Am Acad Child Adolesc Psychiatry 2012;51:192–201.

6. Deckersbach T, Chou T, Britton JC, et al. Neural correlates of behavior therapy for Tourette's disorder. Psychiatry Res 2014;224:269–74.

7. Conelea CA, Woods DW. The influence of contextual factors on tic expression in Tourette's syndrome: a review. J Psychosom Res 2008;65:487–96.

8. Kraft JT, Dalsgaard S, Obel C, et al. Prevalence and clinical correlates of tic disorders in a community sample of school-age children. Eur Child Adolesc Psychiatry 2012;21:5–13.

9. Leckman JF, Zhang H, Vitale A, et al. Course of tic severity in Tourette syndrome: the first two decades. Pediatrics 1998;102:14–9.

10. Mathews CA, Herrera Amighetti LD, Lowe TL, et al. Cultural influences on diagnosis and perception of Tourette syndrome in Costa Rica. J Am Acad Child Adolesc Psychiatry 2001;40:456–63.

11. Leckman JF, Walker DE, Cohen DJ. Premonitory urges in Tourette's syndrome. Am J Psychiatry 1993;150:98–102.

12. Woods DW, Piacentini J, Himle MB, et al. Premonitory Urge for Tics Scale (PUTS): initial psychometric results and examination of the premonitory urge phenomenon in youths with tic disorders. J Dev Behav Pediatr 2005;26:397–403.

13. Scahill L, Aman MG, McDougle CJ, et al. Trial design challenges when combining medication and parent training in children with pervasive developmental disorders. J Autism Dev Disord 2009;39:720–9.

14. Specht MW, Woods DW, Piacentini J, et al. Clinical characteristics of children and adolescents with a primary tic disorder. J Dev Phys Disabil 2011;23:15–31.

15. Bloch MH, Peterson BS, Scahill L, et al. Adulthood outcome of tic and obsessive-compulsive symptom severity in children with Tourette syndrome. Arch Pediatr Adolesc Med 2006;160:65–9.

16. Leckman JF, Riddle MA, Hardin MT, et al. The Yale Global Tic Severity scale: initial testing of a clinician-rated scale of tic severity. J Am Acad Child Adolesc Psychiatry 1989;28:566–73.

17. Cloes KI, Barfell KSF, Horn PS, et al. Preliminary evaluation of child self-rating using the Child Tourette Syndrome Impairment Scale. Dev Med Child Neurol 2017; 59:284–90.

18. Stiede JT, Alexander JR, Wellen B, et al. Differentiating tic-related from non-tic-related impairment in children with persistent tic disorders. Compr Psychiatry 2018;87:38–45.

19. Storch EA, Lack CW, Simons LE, et al. A measure of functional impairment in youth with Tourette's syndrome. J Pediatr Psychol 2007;32:950–9.

20. Hirschtritt ME, Lee PC, Pauls DL, et al. Lifetime prevalence, age of risk, and genetic relationships of comorbid psychiatric disorders in Tourette syndrome. JAMA Psychiatry 2015;72:325–33.

21. Lebowitz ER, Motlagh MG, Katsovich L, et al. Tourette syndrome in youth with and without obsessive compulsive disorder and attention deficit hyperactivity disorder. Eur Child Adolesc Psychiatry 2012;21:451–7.

22. Sambrani T, Jakubovski E, Muller-Vahl KR. New insights into clinical characteristics of Gilles de la Tourette syndrome: findings in 1032 patients from a single German center. Front Neurosci 2016;10:415.
23. Kurlan R, Como PG, Miller B, et al. The behavioral spectrum of tic disorders: a community-based study. Neurology 2002;59.
24. Debes N, Hjalgrim H, Skov L. The presence of attention-deficit hyperactivity disorder (ADHD) and obsessive-compulsive disorder worsen psychosocial and educational problems in Tourette syndrome. J Child Neurol 2010;25:171–81.
25. Eapen V, Črnčec R, McPherson S, et al. Tic disorders and learning disability: clinical characteristics, cognitive performance and comorbidity. Australas J Spec Educ 2013;37:162–72.
26. Eapen V, Cavanna AE, Robertson MM. Comorbidities, social impact, and quality of life in Tourette syndrome. Front Psychiatry 2016;7:97.
27. Barnea M, Benaroya-Milshtein N, Gilboa-Sechtman E, et al. Subjective versus objective measures of tic severity in Tourette syndrome: the influence of environment. Psychiatry Res 2016;242:204–9.
28. Caurín B, Serrano M, Fernández-Alvarez E, et al. Environmental circumstances influencing tic expression in children. Eur J Paediatr Neurol 2014;18:157–62.
29. Bodeck S, Lappe C, Evers S. Tic-reducing effects of music in patients with Tourette's syndrome: self-reported and objective analysis. J Neurol Sci 2015;352:41–7.
30. Silva RR, Munoz DM, Barickman J, et al. Environmental factors and related fluctuation of symptoms in children and adolescents with Tourette's disorder. J Child Psychol Psychiatry 1995;36:305–12.
31. Himle MB, Capriotti MR, Hayes LP, et al. Variables associated with tic exacerbation in children with chronic tic disorders. Behav Modif 2014;38:163–83.
32. Capriotti MR, Piacentini JC, Himle MB, et al. Assessing environmental consequences of ticcing in youth with chronic tic disorders: the Tic Accommodation and Reactions Scale. Child Health Care 2015;44:205–20.
33. Watson TS, Sterling HE. Brief functional analysis and treatment of a vocal tic. J Appl Behav Anal 1998;31:471–4.
34. Eaton CK, Jones AM, Gutierrez-Colina AM, et al. The influence of environmental consequences and internalizing symptoms on children's tic severity. Child Psychiatry Hum Dev 2017;48:327–34.
35. Kim S, Greene DJ, Robichaux-Viehoever A, et al. Tic suppression in children with recent-onset tics predicts 1-year tic outcome. J Child Neurol 2019;34:757–64.
36. Murphy TK, Lewin AB, Storch EA, et al. Practice parameter for the assessment and treatment of children and adolescents with tic disorders: Committee on Quality Issues (CQI). J Am Acad Child Adolesc Psychiatry 2013;52:1341–9.
37. Verdellen C, Van De Griendt J, Hartmann A, et al. European clinical guidelines for Tourette syndrome and other tic disorders. Part III: Behavioural and psychosocial interventions. Eur Child Adolesc Psychiatry 2011;20:197–207.
38. Martino D, Pringsheim TM. Tourette syndrome and other chronic tic disorders: an update on clinical management. Expert Rev Neurother 2018;18:125–37.
39. Pringsheim T, Okun MS, Müller-Vahl K, et al. Practice guideline recommendations summary: treatment of tics in people with Tourette syndrome and chronic tic disorders. Neurology 2019;92:896–906.
40. Weisman H, Qureshi IA, Leckman JF, et al. Systematic review: pharmacological treatment of tic disorders—efficacy of antipsychotic and alpha-2 adrenergic agonist agents. Neurosci Biobehav Rev 2013;37:1162–71.

41. Quezada J, Coffman KA. Current approaches and new developments in the pharmacological management of Tourette syndrome. CNS Drugs 2018;32:33–45.
42. Ross MS, Moldofsky H. A comparison of pimozide and haloperidol in the treatment of Gilles de la Tourette's syndrome. Am J Psychiatry 1978;135:585–7.
43. Shapiro AK, Shapiro E. Controlled study of pimozide vs. placebo in Tourette's syndrome. J Am Acad Child Psychiatry 1984;23:161–73.
44. Shapiro E, Shapiro AK, Fulop G, et al. Controlled study of haloperidol, pimozide, and placebo for the treatment of Gilles de la Tourette's syndrome. Arch Gen Psychiatry 1989;46:722–30.
45. Budman CL. The role of atypical antipsychotics for treatment of Tourette's syndrome: an overview. Drugs 2014;74:1177–93.
46. Roessner V, Plessen KJ, Rothenberger A, et al. European clinical guidelines for Tourette syndrome and other tic disorders. Part II: pharmacological treatment. Eur Child Adolesc Psychiatry 2011;20:173–96.
47. Huys D, Hardenacke K, Poppe P, et al. Update on the role of antipsychotics in the treatment of Tourette syndrome. Neuropsychiatr Dis Treat 2012;8:95–104.
48. Chen JJ, Ondo WG, Dashtipour K, et al. Tetrabenazine for the treatment of hyperkinetic movement disorders: a review of the literature. Clin Ther 2012;34: 1487–504.
49. Jankovic J. Dopamine depleters in the treatment of hyperkinetic movement disorders. Expert Opin Pharmacother 2016;17:2461–70.
50. Kenney C, Hunter C, Jankovic J. Long-term tolerability of tetrabenazine in the treatment of hyperkinetic movement disorders. Mov Disord 2007;22:193–7.
51. Deeb W, Rossi PJ, Porta M, et al. The international deep brain stimulation registry and database for Gilles de la Tourette syndrome: how does it work? Front Neurosci 2016;10:170.
52. Rossi PJ, Opri E, Shute JB, et al. Scheduled, intermittent stimulation of the thalamus reduces tics in Tourette syndrome. Parkinsonism Relat Disord 2016;29: 35–41.
53. Whiting PF, Wolff RF, Deshpande S, et al. Cannabinoids for medical use: a systematic review and meta-analysis. JAMA 2015;313:2456–73.
54. Tourette Association of America position statement on the use of medical marijuana for Tourette Syndrome. Tourette Association of America; 2019. Available at: https://tourette.org/research-medical/medical-marijuana/. Accessed October 25, 2019.
55. Azrin NH, Nunn RG. Habit-reversal: a method of eliminating nervous habits and tics. Behav Res Ther 1973;11:619–28.
56. Azrin NH, Peterson AL. Treatment of Tourette syndrome by habit reversal: a waiting-list control group comparison. Behav Ther 1990;21:305–18.
57. Bate KS, Malouff JM, Thorsteinsson ET, et al. The efficacy of habit reversal therapy for tics, habit disorders, and stuttering: a meta-analytic review. Clin Psychol Rev 2011;31:865–71.
58. McGuire JF, Piacentini J, Brennan EA, et al. A meta-analysis of behavior therapy for Tourette syndrome. J Psychiatr Res 2014;50:106–12.
59. Woods DW, Miltenberger RG. A review of habit reversal with childhood habit disorders. Educ Treat Children 1996;19:197–214.
60. Steeves T, McKinlay BD, Gorman D, et al. Canadian guidelines for the evidence-based treatment of tic disorders: behavioural therapy, deep brain stimulation, and transcranial magnetic stimulation. Can J Psychiatry 2012;57:144–51.

61. Woods DW, Piacentini JC, Chang SW, et al. Managing Tourette syndrome: a behavioral intervention for children and adults. New York: Oxford University Press; 2008.
62. Piacentini J, Woods DW, Scahill L, et al. Behavior therapy for children with Tourette disorder: a randomized controlled trial. J Am Med Assoc 2010;303:1929–37.
63. Woods DW, Piacentini JC, Scahill L, et al. Behavior therapy for tics in children: acute and long-term effects on psychiatric and psychosocial functioning. J Child Neurol 2011;26:858–65.
64. Rizzo R, Pellico A, Silvestri PR, et al. A randomized controlled trial comparing behavioral, educational, and pharmacological treatments in youths with chronic tic disorder or Tourette syndrome. Front Psychiatry 2018;9:100.
65. Hoogduin K, Verdellen C, Cath D. Exposure and response prevention in the treatment of Gilles de la Tourette's syndrome: four case studies. Clin Psychol Psychother 1997;4:125–35.
66. Verdellen CWJ, Keijsers GPJ, Cath DC, et al. Exposure with response prevention versus habit reversal in Tourette's syndrome: a controlled study. Behav Res Ther 2004;42:501–11.
67. Himle MB, Freitag M, Walther M, et al. A randomized pilot trial comparing videoconference versus face-to-face delivery of behavior therapy for childhood tic disorders. Behav Res Ther 2012;50:565–70.
68. Woods DW, Conelea CA, Himle MB. Behavior therapy for Tourette's disorder: utilization in a community sample and an emerging area of practice for psychologists. Prof Psychol Res Pract 2010;41:518–25.
69. Conelea CA, Wellen BCM. Tic treatment goes tech: a review of TicHelper.com. Cogn Behav Pract 2017;24:374–81.
70. Tourette syndrome behavior therapy institute (TS-BTI). Tourette Association of America; 2019. Available at: https://tourette.org/cbit-bti-training/. Accessed October 25, 2019.
71. Sukhodolsky DG, Woods DW, Piacentini J, et al. Moderators and predictors of response to behavior therapy for tics in Tourette syndrome. Neurology 2017;88: 1029–36.
72. Nissen JB, Partner ET, Thomsen PH. Predictors of therapeutic treatment outcome in adolescent chronic tic disorders. BJPsych Open 2019;5:1–6.
73. Deckersbach T, Rauch S, Buhlmann U, et al. Habit reversal versus supportive psychotherapy in Tourette's disorder: a randomized controlled trial and predictors of treatment response. Behav Res Ther 2006;44:1079–90.
74. Peterson BS, Skudlarski P, Anderson AW, et al. A functional magnetic resonance imaging study of tic suppression in Tourette syndrome. Arch Gen Psychiatry 1998;55:326–33.
75. Himle MB, Woods DW. An experimental evaluation of tic suppression and the tic rebound effect. Behav Res Ther 2005;43:1443–51.

Pediatric Prevention
Sleep Dysfunction

Patrick C. Friman, PhD*, Connie J. Schnoes, PhD

KEYWORDS

- Sleep • Children • Bedtime resistance • Night wakings • Insomnia • Parasomnias

KEY POINTS

- Sleep is essential to the healthy growth and development of children and is often overlooked by parents and pediatricians as a contributing factor to concerns for daytime functioning and medical conditions.
- Sleep problems, including delayed sleep onset, night wakings, and bedtime resistance are among the most prevalent concerns reported by caregivers.
- Pediatricians are ideally situated to provide psychoeducation for the prevention and treatment of sleep disorders.

Sleep plays an essential role in the healthy growth and development of children and yet it is often overlooked by caregivers and underemphasized by primary medical providers (pediatricians hereafter). This is partly because the detriments caused by sleep deprivation are not immediately apparent. It is also partly due to a reportedly limited confidence many pediatricians have in their ability to diagnose and treat sleep problems in children.[1] This article addresses the critical role of sleep in the health and functioning of children, describes sleep processes and architecture, and provides information central to identifying and addressing sleep concerns and disorders. Its primary purpose is to serve the pediatrician faced with children at risk for sleep-related problems.

SLEEP MATTERS

Sleep disorders and common sleep problems result in sleep deprivation and or impaired sleep quality and negatively impact the functioning of children and adolescents in myriad ways.[2–8] These deleterious effects are a result of the cumulative nature of sleep deprivation.[9] As an example, a child who sleeps an hour less than recommended nightly for his or her age will have lost nearly an entire night of sleep in 1 week. Deficits of this sort are a regular part of the lives of millions of children and adolescents across this country.[2,10–12]

Center for Behavioral Health, 13460 Walsh Drive, Boys Town, NE 68010, USA
* Corresponding author.
E-mail address: Patrick.friman@boystown.org

Pediatr Clin N Am 67 (2020) 559–571
https://doi.org/10.1016/j.pcl.2020.02.010
0031-3955/20/© 2020 Elsevier Inc. All rights reserved.

The brain and body function differently during sleep than during wakefullness.[13] The central nervous system along with virtually all the other regulatory systems (eg, circulatory, respiratory, endocrine) are actively engaged in restorative processes during sleep. As sleep deprivation increases, restoration declines. Just a few examples of the many critical activities that occur during sleep include release of growth hormone, decreases in cortisol secretion, consolidation of long-term memories, and facilitation of subsequent cognitive and motor performance.

Insufficient total sleep time and impaired sleep quality interfere with sleep-dependent processes. Research with children who present with insufficient or impaired sleep has revealed increased emotional problems,[2,12] poorer school performance,[2,12,14–16] anxiety,[17] increased difficult behaviors,[18–21] poorer cognitive functioning,[21–23] inattention, heightened activity and impulsivity,[24,25] poor concentration,[8] increased risk for obesity,[26,27] decreased general memory,[28,29] more difficult temperament,[30–32] impaired motor skills,[33] more frequent medical attention due to accidents,[34] and increased health problems.[12,35–37]

SLEEP PROCESSES
Biological

Sleep is comprised of 2 sleep states: rapid eye movement (REM) sleep and non-REM sleep. During a night's sleep, children cycle between non-REM sleep, REM sleep, and brief periods of wakefulness. Non-REM sleep occurs in 4 stages of increasing depth as reflected by decreasing electroencephalographic activity. Stage IV, often referred to as delta, is the most restorative stage and also the location of some sleep disorders to be discussed below. Delta sleep gradually decreases over the lifespan as reflected by the depth of sleep in young children and shallowness of sleep in the elderly. Dreaming occurs during REM sleep. The length of the sleep cycle (the time between falling asleep and the first brief awakening) increases from approximately 50 minutes in children to 90 minutes in adolescents.

Two biological processes work in tandem and control the sleep/wake cycle: the homeostatic sleep drive and the circadian rhythm. The homeostatic sleep drive produces increased pressure to sleep in response to being awake over time. The circadian rhythm refers to the central nervous system's governance over wakefulness and sleepiness at different times during the 24-hour day. The homeostatic drive and the circadian system align at night to promote sleep. As the homeostatic drive for sleep decreases during the night the circadian system maintains sleep to allow for attainment of sufficient total sleep time.

Contextual

Falling asleep is a learned process that begins in infancy. Learning to achieve independent sleep induction is necessary for healthy sleep practices.[38] This is accomplished when the child's environment is conducive to independent sleep onset as biological sleep pressure mounts. Putting children to bed sleepy but awake in a sleep-conducive environment (ie, quiet, dark) facilitates this process. When this occurs, the child establishes sleep onset association cues for independent sleep induction. Sleep induction occurs at the end of each sleep cycle throughout the night. When independent sleep induction is established children wake briefly at the end of the sleep cycle and resume sleep independently.

Although independent sleep induction is a critical developmental goal, children often form sleep onset associations that maintain dependent sleep induction. Common sleep onset associations include being rocked or fed to sleep in infants, rocking and/or caregiver presence in toddlers and children, and music, reading, TV, cell phone activities, and so forth, in children and adolescents.[9] When these sleep onset associations are absent, children struggle to fall asleep or resume sleep after waking.

Infants experience rapid changes in their sleep/wake patterns and sleep physiology. In newborns, periods of sleep and wake occur randomly throughout the day and night. By 6 weeks of age, most infants exhibit a clear diurnal/nocturnal pattern of sleep and wake with a clear differentiation of day and night at 3 months and consolidated nighttime sleep by 9 months of age. These rapid changes combined with the infant's inability to settle independently may make it difficult for caregivers to correctly interpret their babies' sleepiness cues. Understanding the basic rest and activity cycle or BRAC may assist caregivers in teaching their babies independent sleep induction skills.[39] Babies initially experience sleep pressure after 90 minutes of wakefulness and need caregiver assistance to fall asleep. Monitoring the baby's wake time, anticipating cues for sleepiness 75 to 90 minutes later, and assisting the baby in falling asleep by decreasing stimulation and helping the baby settle set the stage for independent sleep induction. As babies develop, their periods of wakefulness increase, and they are able settle to sleep independently. The critical facets for caregiver's are the recognition of their babies' sleep cues and their proper response to those cues to promote independent sleep induction.[40]

SLEEP DISORDERS

Most sleep disorders exhibited by children and adolescents fall into 2 categories: dysomnias and parasomnias. Dysomnias interfere with the onset or process of sleep. Parasomnias disrupt sleep once sleep onset has occurred. Difficulty falling asleep and staying asleep and sleeping at inappropriate times of day are characteristic of dysomnias. Manifesting behavior suggestive of wakefulness while simultaneously being asleep is characteristic of parasomnias. For this reason, they are usually referred to as partial arousal parasomnias; that is, the child appears to be partially awake. Most parasomnias occur within the first third of the sleep cycle in conjunction with the transition from delta sleep to lighter sleep stages. The sleep disorders addressed herein are listed below. The diagnostic criteria are taken from the *Diagnostic and Statistical Manual of Mental Disorders* (Fifth Edition) (*DSM-5*)[41] and the *International Classification of Sleep Disorders*.[42]

Dysomnias

- Insomnia
- Circadian rhythm sleep–wake disorder
- Breathing-related sleep disorder
- Narcolepsy

Parasomnias

- Sleep terrors
- Sleepwalking
- Sleep-related eating
- Nightmare disorder
- Rhythmic movement disorder

Insomnia

Insomnia is characterized by difficulty falling asleep, difficulty remaining asleep, or the failure to feel rested after sleeping. Diagnostic criteria require the problem to be present for at least 1 month.[41,42] Difficulty falling asleep or remaining asleep may be associated with many variables. In young children, caregivers most often report bedtime resistance.[43] Bedtime resistance is characterized by reluctance to go to bed and/or stay in bed. Children may dawdle or tantrum during the bedtime routine thus delaying bedtime. Once in bed, children may come out or call out repeatedly resulting in delayed sleep onset before falling asleep on their own.

Insomnia may also manifest in children with dependent sleep onset associations when they are expected to fall asleep independently. These children often engage in a variety of behaviors that are incompatible with sleep onset (eg, calling out, coming out, crying, playing) until the conditions for sleep onset are met. These children are at significant risk for extended night wakings.

Insomnia may also be associated with anxiety or nighttime fears. Some children and adolescents have difficulty falling asleep due to ruminating about past or future events. This rumination makes it difficult to fall asleep. Youth who present with nighttime fears may resist falling asleep to avoid the experience of nightmares or nighttime fears. When children wake from a nightmare, they may have difficulty returning to sleep due to the emotional arousal associated with the nightmare (eg, anxiety).

Circadian Rhythm Sleep–Wake Disorder

Circadian rhythm sleep–wake disorder: delayed sleep phase type is characterized by a consistent and persistent pattern of late sleep onset and late morning awakening times.[41,42] Individuals who present with sleep phase delay are unable to fall asleep at earlier more appropriate times. This disorder is particularly prevalent in adolescents.

Adolescents who present with delayed sleep phase often struggle to awaken in time for early morning activities (eg, school, work, extracurriculars). When they do wake in time for activities, they are at high risk for subsequently falling asleep or exhibiting excessive sleepiness. The problematic effects of delayed sleep phase extend beyond sleep. They also include problems, such as conflict with caregivers, poor school attendance, and impaired academic performance.[8,9]

Breathing-Related Sleep Disorder

Breathing-related sleep disorder: obstructive sleep apnea hypopnea involves obstruction of the airway while asleep resulting in insomnia and excessive daytime sleepiness.[41,42] This disorder affects 1% to 2% of children.[41] Diagnosis of obstructive sleep apnea typically includes an overnight sleep study during which a polysomnography is conducted. This sleep study records the frequency of apneas (the child stops breathing), hypopneas (abnormally slow or shallow breathing) and hypoventilation (abnormal blood oxygen and carbon dioxide levels). When the apneas the child exhibits result in insufficient oxygen levels, the child is diagnosed with obstructive sleep apnea. Children who present with obstructive sleep apnea hypopnea may also exhibit snoring, labored breathing while asleep, daytime mouth breathing, and unusual postures while sleeping. In children, the most common causes of obstruction are enlarged tonsils and or adenoids.

Narcolepsy

Narcolepsy is characterized by irresistible attacks of sleepiness during the daytime. Diagnostic criteria specify that they occur at least 3 times per week over the course of 3 consecutive months.[41,42] Diagnostic criteria also require hypocretin deficiency, rapid onset REM sleep, or cataplexy (sudden bilateral loss of muscle tone for brief episodes often triggered by intense emotional expression).[41,42] In children loss of muscle tone may consist of global hypotonia or grimaces or jaw opening episodes with tongue thrusting in the absence of an emotional trigger.[41] Rapid onset REM sleep is assessed with a multiple sleep latency test and diagnosis requires 2 or more sleep onset REM periods (fall directly into REM sleep).[42] The events typically last for 10 to 20 minutes (although undisturbed the child may sleep up to an hour) and occur 2 to 6 times per day. Narcolepsy is more common among adolescents than younger children.

Parasomnias

Sleep terrors

Sleep terrors, also commonly known as night terrors, affect people of all ages but are most prevalent in young children. Sleep terrors are characterized by an abrupt disruption of sleep approximately 3 hours after falling asleep with the child screaming and crying uncontrollably for 1 to 10 minutes. Diagnostic criteria also include a presentation of appearing fearful, autonomic arousal (tachycardia, rapid breathing, sweating, shaking), unresponsiveness to efforts to wake or comfort, and amnesia for the event.[41]

Sleep terrors are disturbing for caregivers but not for the children themselves. The children are deeply asleep. But their screams and crying wake their caregivers who, when uninformed about night terrors interpret the episode as evidence of extreme child distress. Their subsequent attempts to soothe the child are usually met with resistance and largely fail. Typically, after a few minutes the child quiets and resumes sleeping.

Sleepwalking

Sleepwalking is characterized by getting out of bed and walking or engaging in other complex motor behaviors (running, jumping, navigating stairs, doorways and furniture, urinating, sleep talking) while asleep.[41,42] Children may also appear to be trying to escape something while they are sleepwalking. Children typically return to bed without fully awakening and resume sleep. The child may settle somewhere other than bed and sleep till morning. Diagnostic criteria also include: blank staring, unresponsiveness to others, amnesia for the event, and no impairment of mental or behavioral activity within a few minutes of awakening. Sleepwalking events typically occur toward the end of the first third of the night's sleep period.

Sleepwalking may be instigated by internal states, such as a full bladder or external stimuli, such as ambient noise or movement. Sleepwalking puts children at significantly increased risk for nocturnal accidents (eg, falling down stairs).

Sleep-Related Eating

Sleep-related eating is included as a specifier for sleepwalking in *DSM-5*. Sleep-related eating includes eating during partial arousal from sleep at least 1 time per week.[41] Amnesia for the episode is also a diagnostic criterion. Persons with sleep-related eating usually leave revealing evidence (eg, partially eaten food, crumbs) that an episode has occurred. Afflicted youth usually eat high-calorie foods during the episode. The most significant risk posed by this disorder involves the types of foods eaten during an episode (eg, raw bacon) bizarre preparation of food (eg, cooking, putting jellied bread or raw bacon in a toaster) and the impact on diet, especially for youth with diabetes or those who are overweight. Sleep-related eating is most prevalent in adolescence.

Nightmare Disorder

Nightmare disorder is characterized by the repeated occurrence of extended, extremely upsetting, vivid dreams that typically include threats to survival, safety, or physical danger.[41] Nightmare disorder differs from other parasomnias in 2 significant ways. First, nightmares usually occur at the end of the sleep phase, whereas the other parasomnias usually occur during the first third. Second, those afflicted are able to recall at least some of the content of the episode while the content of the other parasomnias is lost to memory.

Rhythmic Movement Disorder

Rhythmic movement disorder (RMD) is most prevalent in infants and young children. It is characterized by repetitive rhythmic movement (eg, rocking, head banging, swaying) during sleep onset.[42] RMD is diagnosed only if the movement results in injury or interferes with sleep. Prevalence estimates range from 2% to 8% of children.[42] Rhythmic movement in general, however, is very prevalent (ie, 60% percent at 9 months, 33% at 18 months, and 5% at 5 years).[42]

PSYCHOEDUCATION FOR PREVENTION OF SLEEP PROBLEMS

Sleep problems are among the most common reported caregiver concerns in pediatric practice[44] with 30% of caregivers reporting sleep concerns.[45] Up to 40% of children and adolescents exhibit a sleep disorder during their lifetime.[12,17,37,46,47] Furthermore, most sleep problems do not spontaneously resolve.[18,48–50] Pediatricians are in an ideal position to provide psychoeducation that increases awareness of the importance of sleep and promotes healthy sleep behavior. Whether responding to reported sleep concerns or assessing the role of sleep in other reported medical concerns, pediatricians can provide caregivers and patients with information that promotes healthy functioning. Several key variables that facilitate healthy sleep practices are discussed below. These include recommended total sleep time, sleep hygiene, the bedtime routine, the bedroom environment, and transition objects.

Recommended Total Sleep Time

The first step in helping children achieve sufficient total sleep time is learning how much sleep they need and when. This information is optimally delivered during well-child visits. Important topics include optimal sleep time, night versus day distribution, and the diminishing role of naps. **Table 1** lists recommended total sleep time by age from birth through 17 years. From 17 years on the recommended total sleep time is 9 hours per night with a range of 8.5 to 9.5 hours.[43]

Determining how much sleep a child is obtaining is a perpetual line of inquiry for pediatricians.[9,12,17] Keeping a chart in the child's medical record can guide the related inquiry. This allows pediatricians to share accurate information with caregivers and patients. As they explore the current sleep/wake schedule, pediatricians can assess whether a child is getting sufficient sleep, how much time the child is spending in bed, and when sleep is occurring. When sleep problems are reported, pediatricians can inform caregivers about sleep and establish appropriate expectations (eg, total sleep time, sleep onset latency, brief night wakings). For example, although immediate sleep onset would seem optimal, it is more likely a sign that a child is sleep deprived. Healthy sleep onset latencies range from 15 to 30 minutes.[51] As another example, caregivers may expect children to sleep through the night, whereas normal sleep cycles are punctuated with brief crests into brief periods of partial wakefulness.

Even when sleep problems are not reported, questions pertaining to sleep should populate the pediatrician's interview.[8,9,12,17] Ignorance about the importance of sleep and important features of sleep is epidemic.[47] It is distinctly possible for caregivers to have a child who falls asleep readily, sleeps appropriately through the night, and occasionally naps but is still sleep deprived. Although unlikely, a child with these sleep

Table 1 Recommended total hours of sleep by age				
Age	Total Hours:Minutes	Range (Hours:Minutes)	Day (Hours:Minutes)	No. of Naps
1 wk	16:00	14–18	Varied	Varied
1 mo	14:00	12:30–15:30	Varied	Varied
3 mo	13:00	12:00–14:00	4:30	3–4
6 mo	12:30	11:30–13:30	3:15	2–3
9 mo	12:15	11:15–13:15	2:45	2
12 mo	11:45	11–12:30	1:30–2:30	1–2
18 mo	11:35	11–12:15	2:00	1
2 y	11:30	11–12	1:52	1
3 y	11:15	10:45–11:45	0:00–1:30	0–1
4 y	11:00	10:30–11:30	0:00–1:00	0–1
5 y	10:45	10:15–11:15	0	0
6 y	10:30	10–11	0	0
7 y	10:22	9:52–10:52	0	0
8 y	10:15	9:45–10:45	0	0
9 y	10:08	9:35–10:35	0	0
10 y	10:00	9:30–10:30	0	0
11 y	9:52	9:11–10:11	0	0
12 y	9:45	9:15–10:15	0	0
13 y	9:35	9:08–10:08	0	0
14 y	9:30	9:00–10:00	0	0
15 y	9:15	8:45–9:45	0	0
16 y	9:08	8:35–9:35	0	0
17 y	9:00	8:30–9:30	0	0

Data from Ferber R. Solve your child's sleep problems: new revised and expanded edition. New York: Simon and Schuster; 2006.

habits can still fall short of optimal sleep time if caregivers do not know how much to expect. In addition, a child's sleep quality may be impaired by snoring or other sleep disruptions that may have important implications for the child's health.

When a child is achieving insufficient total sleep time, it is best to prescribe gradual increases.[52,53] This can be achieved by setting an earlier bedtime or a later morning wake time. How to increase total sleep time is a decision best made jointly by the child's caregiver and the pediatrician. If earlier bedtime is selected, the caregiver should be instructed to start bedtime a short time earlier (eg, 15 minutes earlier) for a few nights (eg, 3). When the child is falling asleep within 20 minutes, the bedtime can be moved again and this process continues until the optimal sleep amount is obtained. There is 1 caveat, specifically, starting too early may result in the child lying in bed awake for extended periods.

Sleep Hygiene

The cardinal rule of sleep hygiene for children is that the sole purpose of their bed is sleep.[9] Children who violate this rule (eg, reading, videos, TV, gaming, social media) are at heightened risk for sleep problems. Sleep assessment should include all pre- and post-bedtime activities. Sleep interventions should remove all activities not functionally related to the induction of sleep. Additional rules include avoiding strenuous exercise and caffeine intake within an hour or 2 of bedtime, following a regular sleep/wake schedule, and establishing a sleep-conducive bedtime routine and bedroom environment.[9]

Bedtime Routines

A healthy bedtime routine is one whose properties increase sleep pressure. Beyond facilitating sleep, bedtime routines can also supply positive interaction time between caregivers and younger children. The general rules for establishing bedtime routines are (1) keep the routine as consistent as possible; (2) ensure that all activities in the routine increase sleep pressure (ie, conduct routine just before bedtime; put on pajamas or clothes reserved for sleeping); and (3) ensure the routine culminates with the child falling asleep independently. There are some special considerations for infants. Specifically, bottle-feeding should occur before the infant is placed in bed. Once fed the child should be placed in bed sleepy but awake.

Bedroom Environment

The bedroom environment is also an important consideration for teaching healthy sleep habits. An optimal sleep-conducive bedroom environment is quiet with low or no lighting. Low light is defined as insufficient light to read a book. Exposure to sunlight can extend sleep onset latency and promote early morning wakings. Blocking out sunlight with curtains is helpful. White noise can help achieve quiet by covering other sounds and reducing stimulation for the child. The basic point is that a sleep-conducive environment increases sleep pressure, which, in turn, is necessary for learning independent sleep induction and attaining quality sleep.

Transition Objects

To achieve independent sleep induction children must be able to self soothe or reduce arousal. Preferred attachment objects (eg, blanket, stuffed animal, pacifier) can help children achieve these goals. When objects are paired with bedtime and falling asleep they help children independently transition from being awake to being asleep.[9] Transition objects also aid children in resuming sleep independently after night wakings.[54]

COMMON SLEEP CONCERNS

Common presenting sleep concerns include bedtime difficulties, night wakings, extended sleep onset latency (insomnia), and irregular sleep/wake schedules.[9,45] Information on these concerns and how to address them follows.

Bedtime Difficulties

Bedtime difficulties most often consist of bedtime resistance. This resistance includes behaviors, such as calling, crying, coming out from bedrooms, and/or playing in bedrooms extensively (eg, 1 or more hours) before falling asleep. Independent sleepers exhibit prolonged resistance and then fall asleep on their own. Dependent sleepers exhibit resistance until a caregiver joins them and aids the transition to sleep.

Night Wakings

As indicated previously, brief partial waking is part of normal cyclical sleep. Independent sleepers wake briefly and return to sleep on their own. There are 2 exceptions to this, however. First, the wakings may be extended if the child has access to stimulating activities or objects. Second, they may be extended if recommended sleep time as been exceeded.

Dependent sleepers are perpetually at risk for extended night wakings. These children have not developed the ability to self soothe and thus are unable to return to sleep independently after wakings have occurred.

INTERVENTIONS FOR COMMON SLEEP PROBLEMS
Extinction

An effective behavioral strategy for bedtime difficulties and night wakings is extinction (ie, cry it out).[37,38,52,55] In an extinction procedure, caregivers put the child in bed at a designated bedtime and ignore the child until a scheduled morning wake time. Children will cry until they fall asleep, thus crying it out. The duration of crying depends on the child's temperament and learning history and can last for several hours. Each subsequent night the duration of crying decreases. Although this method is highly effective, it is controversial and generates little social acceptance.[42]

Graduated Extinction

Graduated extinction is a variation on the cry it out method.[37,52,55,56] Caregivers put the child to bed and ignore the child for a predetermined time interval that gradually increases (eg, 5, 10, 15 min on the first night and up to 45 minutes on night 7). At the end of the specified time interval, the caregiver checks on the child briefly and silently, refraining from picking up, comforting, and interacting with the child.

Positive Routines

Positive routines[37,52,55] combine extinction with a reinforcing bedtime ritual. Caregivers initiate a bedtime routine that includes several quiet activities a short time (eg, 20–30 minutes) before bedtime. During the routine, the caregiver delivers simple instructions and reinforcement for compliance followed by the final instruction to get in bed and go to sleep. If the child is noncompliant during the routine it is terminated, and the child is told the routine is over and it is time to go to bed. A similar response is delivered if the child leaves the bed at any time. Caregivers ignore crying and verbalizations throughout.

Bedtime Fading or Sleep Restriction

Bedtime fading or sleep restriction is used to establish an earlier sleep/wake schedule for children who exhibit an extended sleep onset latency.[37,52,53,55] This procedure matches bedtime with the child's established sleep onset time and controls the morning wake time. When the child falls asleep within 20 minutes of bedtime for 3 nights the bedtime is moved 15 minutes earlier. The process is repeated until the desired bedtime is achieved. Controlling the morning wake time ensures sufficient sleep pressure at bedtime.

The Bedtime Pass

The bedtime pass is another variation on the extinction method.[57–60] This intervention consists of providing the child with a pass (eg, laminated card) at bedtime that the child can exchange for the satisfaction of a single request (eg, drink, hug, bathroom). On using the pass, all subsequent requests are ignored. Research on the pass reveals that its use is accompanied by very little child resistance and high levels of social acceptance.[57,58,60]

Interventions for Insomnia

The first step in addressing insomnia is to insure the youth is not in bed longer than needed to achieve the recommended amount of total sleep time. The second step is to insure that expectations for sleep onset latency and night wakings are reasonable.[9] Merely correcting problems with these procedures can resolve insomnia. Another strategy is to increase sleep pressure. To do so children are instructed to get out of bed when awake approximately 30 minutes after bedtime. They are encouraged to engage in a quiet activity by low light, such as reading, drawing, or writing (no cell phone, TV, videos, or video games) until they feel sleepy. Once sleepy (sleep pressure has increased) they return to bed.

Interventions for Delayed Sleep Phase

Ensuring adolescents do not have access to preferred activities after bedtime is the first step in addressing sleep phase delay. Encouraging caregivers to establish limits and effective consequences may be necessary. When academic or other responsibilities result in sleep phase delay, problem solving how to manage schedules and activities to allow for a healthy sleep/wake schedule may be helpful. Chronotherapy is an effective intervention that shifts the sleep/wake schedule.[61] This intervention is based on a 27-hour day that moves the sleep cycle forward 3 hours every 24 hours until the desired bedtime is achieved. This intervention involves: (1) setting the initial bedtime at the current sleep onset time (eg, 3 AM); (2) waking the adolescent after 8 hours of sleep (eg, 11 AM); and (3) initiating the next sleep cycle 19 hours later (eg, 6 AM). This process is repeated until the scheduled bedtime coincides with the desired bedtime.

Interventions for Partial Arousal Parasomnias

A first step in addressing partial arousal parasomnias is to assess the total sleep time attained by the child. When the child is sleep deprived, the second step is to increase total sleep time. Sleep quality (eg, sleep disruption, airway obstruction) should be assessed and addressed when children who attain sufficient total sleep time present with partial arousal parasomnias. Increasing total sleep time and or addressing concerns related to sleep quality will resolve at least some partial arousal parasomnias. Scheduled awakenings[37,55,62] is another effective intervention. This method involves briefly waking the child 15 minutes before a typical spontaneous awakening. When spontaneous wakings decrease, scheduled awakenings are faded by increasing the time between initial sleep onset and the scheduled awakening in 30-min increments nightly.

SUMMARY

Although child mental health professionals may feel uniquely qualified to address sleep problems, there is no need to allow the problems get that far. All children have a pediatrician (or the equivalent) and few have a mental health provider. Furthermore, whereas there is a certain stigma attached to seeking mental health services, the stigma that attaches to pediatric health services is not seeking them. The upshot is that all children walk through the pediatrician's door and many, possibly even most, are at risk for some type of sleep problem. Therefore, the pediatrician's office is the ideal place to deliver health education about the importance of sleep, its dynamics, and how to correct for sleep problems when they occur. Establishing healthy sleep practices in children is a significant contribution to their health and wellbeing—the 2 most significant goals of pediatric medicine.

DISCLOSURE

The authors have nothing to disclose.

REFERENCES

1. Owens JA. The practice of pediatric sleep medicine: results of a community survey. Pediatrics 2001;108:e51.
2. Asarnow LD, McGlinchey E, Harvey AG. The effects of bedtime and sleep duration on academic and emotional outcomes in a nationally representative sample of adolescents. J Adolesc Health 2014;54(3):350–6.
3. Dinges DF, Pack F, Williams K, et al. Cumulative sleepiness, mood disturbance, and psychomotor vigilance performance decrements during a week of sleep restricted to 4–5 hours per night. Sleep 1997;20:267–77.
4. Link SC, Ancoli-Israel S. Sleep and the teenager. Sleep Res 1995;24:184.
5. Fredriksen K, Rhodes J, Reddy R, et al. Sleepless in Chicago: tracking the effects of adolescent sleep loss during the middle school years. Child Dev 2004;75: 84–95.
6. Roberts RE, Roberts CR, Duong HT. Sleepless in adolescence: prospective data on sleep deprivation, health and functioning. J Adolesc 2009;32:1045–57.
7. Mindell JA, Owens JA. A clinical guide to pediatric sleep: diagnosis and management of sleep problems. Philadelphia: Lippincott, Williams and Wilkins; 2003.
8. Wolfson AR, Carskadon MA. Sleep schedules and daytime functioning in adolescents. Child Dev 1998;69(4):875–87.
9. Owens J, Witmans M. Sleep problems. Curr Probl Pediatr Adolesc Health Care 2004;334:154–79.
10. Carskadon MA, Mindell J, Drake C. Contemporary sleep patterns of adolescents in the USA: results of the 2006 National Sleep Foundation Sleep in America poll. J Sleep Res 2006;5(Suppl 1):1–93.
11. Calamaro CJ, Mason TB, Ratcliffe SJ. Adolescents living the 24/7 lifestyle: effects of caffeine and technology on sleep duration and daytime functioning. Pediatrics 2009;123:e1005–10.
12. Smaldone A, Honig JC, Byrne MW. Sleepless in America: inadequate sleep and relationships to health and well-being of our nation's children. Pediatrics 2007; 119:s29–37.
13. Carskadon MA, Dement WC. Normal human sleep: an overview. In: Kryger MH, Roth T, Dement WC, editors. Principles and practice of sleep medicine. 4th edition. Philadelphia: Elsevier Saunders; 2005. p. 13–23.
14. Drummond SP, Brown GG, Gillin JC, et al. Altered brain response to verbal learning following sleep deprivation. Nature 2000;403:655–7.
15. Spreen O. Prognosis of learning disability. J Consult Clin Psychol 1988;56: 836–42.
16. Eliasson A, King J, Gould B. Association of sleep and academic performance. Sleep Breath 2002;6:45–8.
17. Steinsbekk S, Berg-Nielsen TS, Wichstrøm L. Sleep disorders in preschoolers: prevalence and comorbidity with psychiatric symptoms. J Dev Behav Pediatr 2013;34:633–41.
18. Kelly Y, Kelly J, Sacker A. Changes in bedtime schedules and behavioral difficulties in 7 year old children. Pediatrics 2013;132:e1184–93.
19. Beebe DW. Cognitive, behavioral, and functional consequences of inadequate sleep in children and adolescents. Pediatr Clin North Am 2011;58:649–65.

20. Lam P, Hiscock H, Wake M. Outcomes of infant sleep problems: a longitudinal study of sleep, behavior, and maternal well-being. Pediatrics 2003;111:e203–7. Available at: http://www.pediatrics.org/cgi/content/full/111/3/e203.

21. Beebe DW, Gozal D. Obstructive sleep apnea and the prefrontal cortex: towards a comprehensive model linking nocturnal upper airway obstruction to daytime cognitive and behavioral deficits. J Sleep Res 2002;11:1–16.

22. Dahl RE. The impact of inadequate sleep on children's daytime cognitive function. Semin Pediatr Neurol 1996;3:44–50.

23. Randazzo AC, Muehlbach M, Schweitzer PK, et al. Cognitive function following acute sleep restriction in children ages 10-14. Sleep 1998;21:861–8.

24. Goll JC, Shapiro CM. Sleep disorders presenting as common pediatric problems. CMAJ 2006;174:617–9.

25. Stephens RJ, Chung SA, Jovanovic D, et al. Relationship between polysomnographic sleep architecture and behavior in medication-free children with TS, ADHD, TS and ADHD, and controls. J Dev Behav Pediatr 2013;34:688–96.

26. Padez C, Mourao I, Moreira P, et al. Long sleep duration and childhood overweight/obesity and body fat. Am J Hum Biol 2009;21(3):371–6.

27. Bell JF, Zimmerman FJ. Shortened nighttime sleep duration in early life and subsequent childhood obesity. Arch Pediatr Adolesc Med 2010;164(9):840–5.

28. Steenari MR, Vuontela V, Paavonen EJ, et al. Working memory and sleep in 6- to 13-year-old schoolchildren. J Am Acad Child Adolesc Psychiatry 2003;42(1):85–92.

29. Walker MP, Stickgold R. Sleep, memory, and plasticity. Annu Rev Psychol 2006;57(1):139–66.

30. Carey WB. Night waking and temperament in infancy. Behav Pediatr 1974;84:756–8.

31. Schaefer CE. Night waking and temperament in early childhood. Psychol Rep 1990;67:192–4.

32. Weissbluth M. Sleep duration and infant temperament. J Pediatr 1981;99:817–9.

33. Kuriyama K, Stickgold R, Walker MP. Sleep dependent learning and motor-skill complexity. Learn Mem 2004;11(6):705–13.

34. Koulouglioti C, Cole R, Kitzman H. Inadequate sleep and unintentional injuries in young children. Public Health Nurs 2008;25(2):106–14.

35. Moole S, Singareddy R, Calhoun S, et al. Gastrointestinal symptoms are more common in young school aged children with sleep disturbances. Am J Gastroenterol 2008;103:S531–2.

36. Bryant PA, Trinder J, Curtis N. Sick and tired: does sleep have a vital role in the immune system? Nat Rev Immunol 2004;4(6):457–67.

37. Mindell JA, Kuhn B, Lewin DS, et al. Behavioral treatment of bedtime problems and night wakings in infants and young children. Sleep 2006;29:1263–76.

38. Morrell J, Cortina-Borja M. The developmental change in strategies parents employ to settle young children to sleep, and their relationship to infant sleeping problems, as assessed by a new questionnaire: the parental interactive bedtime behaviour scale. Infant Child Dev 2002;11:17–41.

39. Moore P. The natural baby sleep solution: use your child's internal sleep rhythms for better nights and naps. New York: Workman; 2016.

40. Kerr SM, Jowett SA, Smith LN. Preventing sleep problems in infants: a randomized controlled trial. J Adv Nurs 1996;24:938–42.

41. American Psychiatric Association. In: Diagnostic and statistical manual of mental disorders, Fifth edition (DSM-5). Washington, DC: American Psychiatric Publishing; 2013.

42. American Academy of Sleep Medicine (AASM). The International classification of sleep disorders, diagnostic and coding manual third edition. Westchester (IL): American Academy of Sleep Medicine; 2014.

43. Ferber R. Solve your child's sleep problems: new revised and expanded edition. New York: Simon and Schuster; 2006.

44. Chervin R, Archbold K, Panahi P, et al. Sleep problems seldom addressed in two general pediatric clinics. Pediatrics 2001;107:1375–80.

45. Lozoff B, Wolf AW, Davis NS. Sleep problems seen in pediatric practice. Pediatrics 1985;75:477–83.

46. Meltzer LJ, Mindell JA. Sleep, sleep disorders in children and adolescents. Pediatr Clin North Am 2006;29:1059–76.

47. National Sleep Foundation. Sleep in America poll. Washington (DC): American Academy of Sleep Medicine; 2006.

48. Zuckerman B, Stevenson J, Bailey V. Sleep problems in early childhood: continuities, predictive factors, and behavioral correlates. Pediatrics 1987;80:664–71.

49. Kataria S, Swanson MS, Trevathon GE. Persistence of sleep disturbances in preschool children. J Pediatr 1987;110:642–6.

50. Pollock JI. Night waking at five years of age: predictors and prognosis. J Child Psychol Psychiatry 1994;35:699–708.

51. Gellis LA, Lichstein KL. Sleep hygiene practices of good and poor sleepers in the United States: an internet-based study. Behav Ther 2009;40:1–9.

52. Friman PC. Behavioral pediatrics: integrating applied behavior analysis with pediatric medicine. In: Fisher W, Piazza C, Roane H, editors. Handbook of applied behavior analysis. 2nd edition, in press.

53. Spielman AJ, Chien-Ming Y, Glovinsky PB. Sleep restriction therapy. In: Perlis M, Aloia M, Kuhn B, editors. Behavioral treatments for sleep disorders: a comprehensive primer of behavioral sleep medicine interventions. London: Elsevier; 2001. p. 9–19.

54. Wolf AW, Lozoff B. Object attachment, thumbsucking and the passage to sleep. J Am Acad Child Adolesc Psychiatry 1989;28:287–92.

55. Mindell JA. Empirically supported treatments in pediatric psychology: bedtime refusal and night wakings in young children. J Pediatr Psychol 1999;24:465–81.

56. Jin CS, Hanley GP, Beaulieu L. An individualized and comprehensive approach to treating sleep problems in young children. J Appl Behav Anal 2013;46:161–80.

57. Friman PC, Hoff KE, Schnoes CJ, et al. The bedtime pass: an approach to bedtime crying and leaving the room. Arch Pediatr Adolesc Med 1999;153:1027–9.

58. Freeman KA. Treating bedtime resistance with bedtime pass: a systematic replication and component analysis with 3-year olds. J Appl Behav Anal 2006;3:423–8.

59. Schnoes CJ. The bedtime pass. In: Perlis M, Aloia M, Kuhn B, editors. Behavioral treatments for sleep disorders: a comprehensive primer of behavioral sleep medicine interventions. Boston: Elsevier; 2011. p. 293–8.

60. Moore BA, Friman PC, Fruzzetti AE, et al. Evaluating the bedtime pass program for child resistance to bedtime: a randomized, controlled trial. J Pediatr Psychol 2007;32:283–7.

61. Czeisler C, Richarson G, Coleman R, et al. Chronotherapy: resetting the circadian clocks of patients with delayed sleep phase insomnia. Sleep 1981;4:1–21.

62. Rickert VI, Johnson CM. Reducing nocturnal awakening and crying episodes in infants and young children: a comparison between scheduled awakenings and systematic ignoring. Pediatrics 1988;81:203–12.

Pediatric Prevention
Teaching Safety Skills

Raymond G. Miltenberger, PhD, BCBA-D[a],*,
Sindy Sanchez, PhD, BCBA-D[b], Diego Valbuena, PhD, BCBA-D[b]

KEYWORDS

- Abduction prevention • Behavioral skills training • Gun safety • In situ assessment
- In situ training • Injury prevention • Safety skills

KEY POINTS

- Exposure to dangerous items (firearms, poisons) or dangerous interactions with adults (abduction attempts) is infrequent and unpredictable but can lead to serious injury and death.
- One approach to prevention is to teach safety skills so children learn to respond appropriately to these safety threats.
- Safety skills consist of identifying, avoiding, escaping, and reporting the safety threat.
- Informational approaches to training that consist of only instructions and modeling are not effective for teaching safety skills.
- Active learning approaches (behavioral skills training and in situ training) are the most effective approaches to training.

INTRODUCTION

In the United States, unintentional injuries are the leading cause of mortality in children, accounting for 44% of deaths in children aged 1–19 years. Preventable causes of injuries and death, which include drowning, burns/fire, transport-related injuries, suffocation, and unintentional firearm injuries, result in the death of approximately 20 children daily.[1] In addition, 9.8 million children receive emergency medical care for unintentional injuries every year.[1]

Unintentional injuries can result from a variety of safety threats. These safety threats can be separated into 2 main categories: (1) frequently occurring (and predictable) threats, and (2) infrequent (and unpredictable) threats.[2,3] Frequently occurring threats present repeated and predictable opportunities to practice safety skills to prevent injuries. For example, safety skills such as the use of protective equipment during

a Department of Child and Family Studies, University of South Florida, MHC2113A, Tampa, FL 33612, USA; b 8209 Bally Money Road, Tampa, FL 33610, USA
* Corresponding author.
E-mail address: miltenbe@usf.edu

Pediatr Clin N Am 67 (2020) 573–584
https://doi.org/10.1016/j.pcl.2020.02.011
0031-3955/20/© 2020 Elsevier Inc. All rights reserved.

sports, helmets while bike riding, or safety restraints when in vehicles are used in predictable circumstances that occur frequently in children's lives. Infrequent but unpredictable safety threats, such as encountering an unattended gun, being in a fire, finding poisonous chemicals, or facing attempted abductions, may be lethal and present limited opportunities to practice the safety skills. This article focuses on the assessment and teaching of safety skills to children to avoid injuries or death from low-probability but highly dangerous safety threats (eg, firearms, poison, abduction).

Note that the responsibility for children's safety lies squarely on the shoulders of adults.[2,3] Many childhood injuries can be prevented through safe practices by adults that reduce or eliminate safety threats. For example, poisoning can be prevented by locking up medicines and toxic chemicals and keeping them out of reach of children. However, this is not always done, because 300 children in the United States are treated for being poisoned every day, with 2 of those children dying.[4] Unintentional firearm injuries can be prevented by safe storage practices by gun owners (eg, keeping firearms in locked safes out of the reach of children). However, this is not always the case, because there were 82 fatal and 1244 nonfatal unintentional firearm injuries between 2012 and 2014.[5]

Although many injuries can be prevented by eliminating the safety threat, children may still encounter safety threats in situations throughout their lives. Therefore, it is imperative to teach children how to respond safely if they encounter a threat such as an unattended firearm, dangerous chemicals, a stranger's lure, or a fire. Although the risks presented by these threats differ, the safety skills for responding to the threats are generally the same. These core safety skills consist of identifying the threat and avoiding contact with it, leaving the area (escaping from the threat), and reporting the threat to a trusted adult or authority figure (**Box 1**).[2]

ASSESSMENT

There are 3 ways to assess the acquisition and generalization of safety skills: verbal report, role play, and in situ assessments.[2,3] In general, children's responses to these assessments are scored using a 0 to 3 rating scale (0 = the child does not demonstrate any of the safety skills; 1 = the child does not interact with the threat but does not leave the area or tell an adult; 2 = the child does not interact with the threat, leaves the area, but does not tell an adult; 3 = the child does not interact with the threat, leaves the area, and tells an adult).

Verbal Report Assessment

In a verbal report assessment, children are presented with a scenario about a safety threat and asked what they would do in that situation.[2,3] For example, the trainer may say, "Imagine you are at home and your dad asks you to get a book from his nightstand. You open the drawer and find a gun. What would you do?" This type of

---

Box 1
Three core safety skills

Identify the safety threat and avoid contact with it

Escape from the threat

Inform an adult about the threat (so the adult can remove it)

assessment indicates the learner's knowledge of, or ability to describe, the safety skills. It does not assess execution of the skills.

Verbal report assessments have been used to evaluate children's knowledge of firearm safety skills,[6–8] fire safety skills,[9] sexual abuse prevention skills,[10–13] and abduction prevention skills.[14,15] Although many of these studies found improvements in responding compared with baseline, not all studies evaluated the children's use of the safety skills during in situ assessments.[11,12] Furthermore, the results of several studies suggest that, although children are able to state the safety skills needed in response to a safety threat, they are unable to demonstrate the safety skills during an a real-life situation.[6,7,14,15] **Fig. 1** shows an example of the low correspondence between verbal report assessment and in situ assessment.

Role-Play Assessment

In a role-play assessment, children are presented with a scenario and asked to act out what they would do in that situation.[6–8] For example, the trainer may place a disabled firearm on a table and say, "Pretend I am your dad and I am watching TV in the other room. I ask you to go to my night table and bring me a book. You find a gun on my night table. Show me what you would do." This type of assessment indicates whether the skills are present in the learner's repertoire.

Unlike verbal report assessments, role-play assessments require active demonstration of the safety skills and are thus a better indication of the safety skills.[2,3] However, role-play assessments do not assess the use of the skills in the natural environment. Three studies compared responses during role-play assessments and in situ assessments for a control group and 2 training groups when finding an unattended firearm.[6–8] The results indicated that children scored higher in role-play assessments than in situ assessments (simulating real-life situations, further discussed later), showing that although children could perform the safety skills in the presence of a trainer, they did not show the safety skills when they were alone in the presence of the simulated but seemingly real safety threat. **Fig. 2** shows an example of the disparity in responding between role-play and in situ assessments.

In Situ Assessment

In an in situ, or in situation, assessment, the child is exposed to a simulated safety threat in the natural environment when the child is unaware of being observed.[2,3] Because research suggests inconsistencies between children's responses to verbal

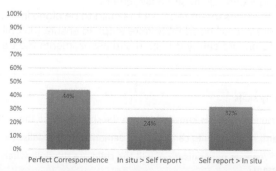

Fig. 1. Correspondence between In situ and Self report Assessment. (*Data from* Carroll-Rowan L, Miltenberger R. A comparison of procedures for teaching abduction prevention to preschoolers. Educ Treat Child 1994;17:113–28.)

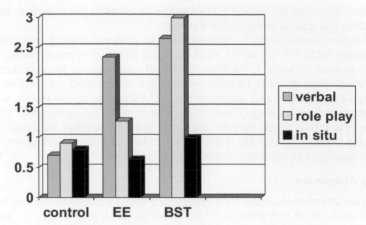

Fig. 2. The group mean scores (0–3 point scale) on verbal report assessment, role-play assessment, and in situ assessment of gun safety skills for each of 3 groups: control, Eddie Eagle GunSafe Program (EE), and behavioral skills training (BST). (*Data from* Himle M, Miltenberger R, Gatheridge B, et al. An evaluation of two procedures for training skills to prevent gun play in children. Pediatrics. 2004;113(1):70-77.)

and role-play assessments and their actions in the presence of a safety threat,[14,16] it is imperative that in situ assessments are conducted without the child's knowledge. In situ assessments assess the generalized use of the safety skills in the natural environment (**Box 2**).

In situ assessments comprise 3 essential features[2,3]:

1. The child encounters a simulated threat in the natural environment (the simulated threat must seem real to the learner).
2. The learner has no knowledge of the assessment or of being observed.
3. An adult is not present when the child encounters the safety threat.

For example, consider how an in situ assessment would be conducted to evaluate the use of gun safety skills by preschool children.[7] To conduct the assessments, the researchers placed a disabled firearm in an unused classroom and a teacher took the child to the classroom to work on a project. When they arrived at the door, the teacher sent the child into the classroom alone and said she would be back in a minute. The child's reaction to finding the gun was recorded on hidden video camera. **Box 3** provides details on conducting an in situ assessment.

Because an in situ assessment requires the child to be alone in the presence of the simulated safety threat, it is important to take steps to ensure the child's safety during the assessment. To ensure safety during in situ assessments the trainer should:

Box 2
Assessment of safety skills

Verbal report assessment. Assesses knowledge: can the child describe the skills?

Role-play assessment. Assesses skills: can the child demonstrate the skills?

In situ assessment.[a] Assesses generalization: will the child use the skills when the (simulated) safety threat is present?

   [a] In situ assessment is the only valid form of assessment of safety skills.

Box 3
Steps for conducting in situ assessments

1. Select the safety threat and identify the corresponding safety responses. Develop a rating scale.

2. The safety threat should seem real but pose no danger (eg, disabled or replica gun).

3. Place the simulated threat in the natural environment ahead of the assessment without the child's knowledge (eg, put a disabled firearm on top of a counter in the kitchen).

4. Make sure the child does not have knowledge of the assessment and does not see the researcher before the assessment.

5. Set up a hidden camera or find a way to view the child without being seen.

6. Make sure the parent (or other trusted adult) is accessible in another room.

7. Have the parent send the child to the room for some valid reason (eg, say "I have a snack for you on the kitchen counter.").

8. The setup should not be an errand, so the child has no expectation of returning immediately.

9. Children should believe they are alone with the safety threat with no one watching.

10. If the child returns to report the gun, provide praise and then go and remove the gun.

11. If the child does not return to report the gun in 30 s, enter the room and remove the gun with no discussion of its presence or the child's behavior.

12. After the assessment, do not debrief the child about the assessment.

---

1. Observe the child continuously throughout the assessment (surreptitiously from nearby or by live video feed).
2. Ensure the parent or teacher is out of sight but within the vicinity of the child
3. Ensure the simulated safety threat cannot harm the child (eg, use only disabled or replica firearms, make sure simulated poisons are inert, make sure lighters are disabled and free of lighter fluid).
4. Ensure the child does not leave the assessment situation (especially important during assessment of abduction prevention skills in a public location).

In situ assessments have been conducted to evaluate children's responses to a variety of safety threats, including abduction lures,[14,15,17,18] finding an unattended firearm,[6,7,19] finding poisonous hazards,[20] and pedestrian safety.[21] Although most of the literature has focused on assessing safety skills by individual children, sometimes children encounter a safety threat in the presence of a peer and, therefore, some researchers have conducted in situ assessments with dyads (**Box 3**).[22–25]

TEACHING SAFETY SKILLS

The literature on teaching safety skills focuses on 2 approaches: informational (passive learning) and active learning.[2,3] The informational or passive approach uses instructions and modeling. The instructor explains the safety threat to the child, tells the child what to do should the child encounter the threat, models the safety skills, and gives the child the opportunity to state what should be done in the presence of a safety threat. In the active learning approach, the instructor incorporates a behavioral rehearsal component during which the child must demonstrate the safety skills so the instructor can praise correct responses and provide corrective feedback for incorrect responses.

Informational Approaches

Informational approaches have been evaluated to teach various safety skills to children, including abduction and sexual abuse prevention and gun safety. One benefit of informational approaches is the ease with which they can be conducted and their adaptability to different instructional modalities, such as in person,[23,24] videos,[18] and workbooks.[13] Some commercially available programs include the Eddie Eagle GunSafe Program,[6,7] the Red Flag Green Flag sexual abuse prevention program,[13,16] and the Stranger Safety abduction prevention program.[18]

The effectiveness of informational approaches has been evaluated using verbal report and in situ assessments. The outcomes of these studies show that informational approaches increase the learner's knowledge of the safety threat and safety skills[6,7] as shown by verbal report assessments. However, research has shown that informational approaches do not result in the use of the safety skills during situ assessments,[6,7,24] and, as such, they are not effective at promoting the acquisition and generalization of safety skills. For example, 2 studies evaluated the Eddie Eagle GunSafe Program, designed to teach children to not touch, get away, and tell an adult when they find a gun.[6,7] The Eddie Eagle program uses instructions, a coloring book, and video modeling but includes no active rehearsal of the skills. This research showed that children participating in the Eddie Eagle program described the safety skills correctly during verbal report assessments but did not show the safety skills during in situ assessments (see **Fig. 2**). Two studies evaluating an informational program designed to teach abduction prevention skills produced similar results.[18,26] Children who watched the Stranger Safety DVD did not engage in the safety skills (run away and tell an adult) during in situ assessments when approached by a stranger. These studies and others show that informational approaches to teaching safety skills are not effective.

Active Learning Approaches

Unlike passive learning approaches that use only instructions and modeling, active learning approaches include rehearsal of the safety skills with feedback.[2,3] In active learning approaches, learners practice the safety skills in the presence of simulated safety threats in role plays or in the natural environment and receive immediate feedback. The main active learning approaches are behavioral skills training (BST) and in situ training (IST).

Behavioral skills training
BST consists of 4 components[2,3]:

1. Instruction: the trainer describes the safety threat and safety skills the child should engage in when presented with that threat
2. Modeling: the trainer demonstrates the safety skills in response to the simulated safety threat, either in person or through video
3. Rehearsal: the trainer requires the learner to practice engaging in the safety skills in response to the simulated safety threat
4. Feedback: the trainer provides praise for correctly demonstrating the safety skills and further instructions on components performed incorrectly

The key components making this an active learning approach are the repeated rehearsals of the safety skills with feedback during role-play scenarios. The practice of the safety skills in the presence of simulated safety threats allows trainers to reinforce correct responses, making the children more likely to engage in the safety skills in response to real-life safety threats similar to those that were simulated during training.

Box 4
Steps for conducting behavioral skills training

Instructions
    Describe the safety threat and why it is dangerous
    Describe the safety skills in context of the safety threat and setting
    Include props (common stimuli) with instructions
    Have the child verbalize the safety skills
    Provide multiple exemplars

Modeling: live or video
    Use a role play to show the safety threat and the safety skills
    Include common stimuli (a disabled or replica firearm)
    Show positive consequences for the model using the safety skills
    Have the learner say what the model did right
    Show multiple exemplars

Rehearsal and feedback
    Have the child rehearse the skills immediately following instructions and modeling
    Describe a role-play scenario with details of the natural environment
    Present simulated safety threat in the role play and ask the child to show what should be done
        Use common stimuli
        Simulate real settings
        Leave the room so the child has to leave the room to find you and report the firearm
    Provide the child the opportunity to demonstrate the safety skills
    Provide immediate feedback
        Praise for correct performance
        Further instruction for improvement
        Repeat until correct
        Provide multiple opportunities for rehearsal and feedback with multiple exemplars

---

Strategies to promote generalization are an important aspect of BST (**Box 5**). The goal is not only to teach safety skills but also to promote their generalization to the natural environments where safety threats occur. Several strategies are used during BST to promote generalization.[3] First, training should include multiple exemplars; that is, all relevant aspects or variations of the safety threat should be incorporated into training. For example, in teaching a safe response to finding a gun, the trainer should conduct training in a variety of different locations in the home where a gun might be found. Second, common stimuli or aspects of the natural environment should be incorporated into training. For example, a trainer should use a real, disabled gun during training so the child is responding in the presence of the same stimulus that should evoke the safety skills in the natural environment. Third, trainers should fade prompts and fade their presence during training trials so the learners are making the correct response in the presence of the simulated safety threat without the stimulus control exerted by prompts or the presence of the trainer. For example, the trainer should ask the child to walk into the room and find the gun alone and then run out of the room to find the adult to report the gun.

BST has been used to teach children a variety of safety skills, including pedestrian safety,[27] fire safety,[28] firearm safety,[6,7,29] abduction prevention,[14,17,30] poison prevention,[20] and sexual abuse prevention.[31] Despite being more effective than informational approaches for teaching safety skills, not all children generalize the safety skills to the natural environment (assessed through in situ assessments) following BST alone. In cases in which BST does not produce generalization of the skills to the natural environment, the addition of in situ training is often successful. The steps involved in conducting BST are shown in **Box 4**.

Box 5
Strategies to promote generalization with behavioral skills training

Include multiple exemplars in training

Include common stimuli in training

Fade prompts and trainer presence before training is finished

---

In situ training

IST follows a failed in situ assessment and consists of a training session in the context in which the safety threat was encountered.[2,3] Following incorrect responding during an in situ assessment, the trainer (who is out of sight) enters the area and immediately turns the failed assessment into a BST session. For example, when a child finds a gun during an in situ assessment but does not engage in the safety skills, the previously unseen trainer (or parent) enters the room, catches the child in the presence of the gun, and requires the child to practice the safety skills multiple times in the situation (eg, run out of the room and tell a parent about the gun). In situ training uses the active learning components of BST and increases generalization of the safety skills as the child is required to engage in the safety skills in the presence of the seemingly real safety threat in the natural environment.

IST has been shown to be successful when used by itself as a stand-alone procedure,[26] following informational approaches,[18,26] and following or combined with BST.[6,17,29,32] IST has been used to teach gun safety skills,[6,29] poisonous hazards prevention,[20] abduction prevention skills,[17,33,34] and fire safety skills.[35]

Gatheridge and colleagues[6] used BST and IST to teach gun safety skills to a group of children 6 and 7 years old. After BST alone was effective for only some of the children (as measured by in situ assessments), the investigators implemented IST. Following IST, all participants demonstrated the gun safety skills during subsequent in situ assessments. Similar results were obtained by Miltenberger and colleagues,[36] who reported that BST alone was only effective for about half of the participants and additional IST sessions were required for safety skills to be shown by all the children. In these studies, IST was used when participants failed to demonstrate the safety skills during in situ assessments following BST. However, Miltenberger and colleagues[29] showed that incorporating IST earlier strengthened the effects of BST for teaching gun safety skills to children. In addition, other investigators have shown the effectiveness of IST as a stand-alone intervention to teach firearm safety skills[22] and abduction prevention skills.[26] The results of these studies suggest that introducing IST earlier in training may result in better generalization of the safety skills and that IST on its own is successful at teaching gun safety and abduction prevention skills to children. The steps involved in conducting IST are shown in **Box 6**.

INCREASING ACCESSIBILITY

Despite being more effective than informational approaches, active learning approaches require more time, effort, and resources from the trainers. Because BST and IST require in-person rehearsal and individualized feedback, researchers have examined avenues to maximize the reach of these interventions by teaching others to conduct training and using simulation training (**Box 7**).

Peers as Trainers

One approach to increase accessibility of safety skills training is the use of peers to implement the trainings. Peer implementation has the benefit of reducing the adult

---

Box 6
Steps for conducting in situ training

1. Conduct an in situ assessment

2. If the child does not show the safety skills in the presence of the safety threat, enter the room

3. Express concern about the safety threat with a serious tone of voice

4. Review the safety skills

5. Require multiple rehearsals on the spot
   Use prompts if needed to get the child to rehearse the skills
   Ignore complaints
   State that the child must get it right before you can be done
   Praise correct rehearsals

6 End with an expectation statement (eg, "If you ever see a gun again, don't touch it; run away, and tell an adult, just like you practiced.")

7. Continue to conduct in situ assessments and IST as needed

8. Add preferred reinforcers for correct performance if needed

Considerations
   IST is always conducted in the context of an in situ assessment
   Never let the child see you before the assessment
   Make sure the in situ assessment is not predicable

---

trainers' involvement while increasing the number of children who receive training. Researchers have used BST to teach older children how to implement BST and IST to teach gun safety skills[32] and abduction prevention skills[37] to younger children. The child trainers successfully implemented BST and IST, and the younger students demonstrated the safety skills during posttraining and follow-up in situ assessments. Furthermore, the child trainers themselves demonstrated the safety skills during in situ assessments.

Parents/Teachers as Trainers

Another approach to increase accessibility of training is to train parents and teachers to teach safety skills. For example, Beck and Miltenberger[18] used an instructional script and protocol followed by modeling, rehearsal, and feedback to teach parents to implement IST to teach their children abduction prevention skills. Gross and colleagues[19] used a manual and video to teach parents to implement BST to teach their children gun safety skills. Carrol-Rowan and Miltenberger[14] used a video or in-person training to train teachers to implement BST to teach preschool children abduction prevention skills. More recently, a Web-based training manual with videos for teaching parents to conduct BST for teaching their children gun safety skills was evaluated (Novotny M, Miltenberger RG. Frederick K, et al. Unpublished manuscript, 2019). In

---

Box 7
Strategies to increase accessibility of safety skills training

Train peers to conduct training

Train parents to conduct training

Use simulation training

---

each of these studies, the parents or teachers successfully implemented training to promote safety skills with their children or students.

Simulation Training

Another potential avenue for increasing accessibility is simulation training. For example, Maxfield and colleagues[38] showed the success of small-scale simulation for teaching firearm safety skills to preschoolers. During the small-scale simulation training, the researchers used BST to teach participants to maneuver a doll to engage in safety skills when encountering a gun in a model house. Similar small-scale simulation trainings have been used to teach pedestrian and transportation skills to individuals with disabilities.[34,39]

Vanselow and Hanley[40] evaluated computerized BST (CBST) for teaching children poison prevention, abduction prevention, and lighter safety skills. CBST included information on safety threats, instructions, video models, and games that incorporated the rehearsal component through simulations. Although only a few participants demonstrated the safety skills following CBST alone, the combination of CBST and IST resulted in the acquisition of the safety skills as well, as generalization to safety skills that were not explicitly trained. When combined with IST, CBST may be a more efficient training alternative to in-person BST.

More recently, Çakiroğlu and Gökoğlu[41] evaluated BST and IST through a virtual reality environment to teach children fire safety skills. The researchers found that children significantly improved their fire safety skills as measured through virtual reality in situ assessments. Furthermore, most children demonstrated the safety skills during in situ assessments. Future research should continue to explore the validity of virtual reality assessments and the effectiveness of active training approaches through virtual reality.

SUMMARY

Threats to child safety, such as abduction attempts, finding unattended firearms, or finding poisons, are unpredictable and infrequent, but potentially deadly. Although it is the responsibility of parents to remove safety threats to keep children safe, some threats will continue to be present so it is valuable to teach safety skills to children. Research shows active learning approaches such as BST and IST are most effective, whereas informational approaches are not. Because children are most at risk from safety threats when they are alone, in situ assessments are the most valid form of assessment because they assess the child's response to a simulated safety threat while alone. BST and IST are the most successful interventions because they provide the opportunity for repeated rehearsals of the skills with reinforcement in the presence of the simulated safety threat and promote generalization of the skills to the natural environment.

DISCLOSURE

The authors have nothing to disclose.

REFERENCES

1. Borse N, Gilchrist J, Dellinger A, et al. CDC childhood injury report: patterns of unintentional injuries among 0-19 year olds in the United States, 2000-2006. Atlanta (GA): US Dept of Health and Human Services; 2008. Available at: http://www.cdc.gov/safechild/images/CDC-ChildhoodInjury.pdf. Accessed July 1, 2019.

2. Miltenberger R, Hanratty L. Teaching sexual abuse prevention skills to children. In: Bromberg D, O'Donohue W, editors. Handbook of child and adolescent sexuality. London: Elsevier Inc; 2013. p. 419–47.

3. Miltenberger R, Sanchez S, Valbuena D. Teaching safety skills to children. In: Roane S, Ringdahl J, Falcomata T, editors. Clinical and organizational applications of applied behavior analysis. London: Elsevier; 2015. p. 477–99.

4. Protect the ONES YOU LOVE: CHILD INJURIES ARE PREventable. CDC.gov. 2016. Available at: https://www.cdc.gov/safechild/poisoning/index.html. Accessed July 20, 2015.

5. Fowler K, Dahlberg L, Haileyesus T, et al. Childhood firearm injuries in the United States. Pediatrics 2017;140(1):e20163486.

6. Gatheridge B, Miltenberger R, Huneke D, et al. Comparison of two programs to teach firearm injury prevention skills to 6-and-7-year old children. Pediatrics 2004;114(3):294–9.

7. Himle M, Miltenberger R, Gatheridge B, et al. An evaluation of two procedures for training skills to prevent gun play in children. Pediatrics 2004;113(1):70–7.

8. Kelso P, Miltenberger R, Waters M, et al. Teaching skills to second and third grade children to prevent gun play: A comparison of procedures. Educ Treat Child 2007;30(3):29–48.

9. Jones RT, Kazdin AE, Haney JI. Social validation and training of emergency fire safety skills for potential injury prevention and life saving. J Appl Behav Anal 1981;14(3):249–60.

10. Harvey P, Forehand R, Brown C, et al. The prevention of sexual abuse: examination of the effectiveness of a program with kindergarten-age children. Behav Ther 1988;19:429–35.

11. Hazzard A, Webb C, Kleemeier C, et al. Child sexual abuse prevention: evaluation and one-year follow-up. Child Abuse Negl 1991;15:123–38.

12. Kenny MC, Wurtele SK, Alonso L. Evaluation of a personal safety program with Latino preschoolers. J Child Sex Abus 2012;21(4):368–85.

13. Miltenberger RG, Thiesse-Duffy E. Evaluation of home-based programs for teaching personal safety skills to children. J Appl Behav Anal 1988;21(1):81–7.

14. Carroll-Rowan L, Miltenberger R. A comparison of procedures for teaching abduction prevention to preschoolers. Educ Treat Child 1994;17:113–28.

15. Olsen-Woods LA, Miltenberger RG, Foreman G. Effects of correspondence training in an abduction prevention training program. Child Fam Behav Ther 1998;20(1):15–34.

16. Miltenberger R, Thiesse-Duffy E, Suda K, et al. Teaching prevention skills to children: The use of multiple measures to evaluate parent versus expert instruction. Child Fam Behav Ther 1990;12:65–87.

17. Johnson BM, Miltenberger RG, Egemo-Helm K, et al. Evaluation of behavioral skills training for teaching abduction-prevention skills to young children. J Appl Behav Anal 2005;38(1):67–78.

18. Beck KV, Miltenberger RG. Evaluation of a commercially available program and in situ training by parents to teach abduction-prevention skills to children. J Appl Behav Anal 2009;42(4):761–72.

19. Gross A, Miltenberger R, Knudson P, et al. Preliminary evaluation of a parent training program to prevent gun play. J Appl Behav Anal 2007;40(4):691–5.

20. Dancho KA, Thompson RH, Rhoades MM. Teaching preschool children to avoid poison hazards. J Appl Behav Anal 2008;41(2):267–71.

21. McComas J, MacKay M, Pivik J. Effectiveness of virtual reality for teaching pedestrian safety. Cyberpsychol Behav 2002;5(3):185–90.

22. Miltenberger R, Gross A, Knudson P, et al. Evaluating behavioral skills training with and without simulated in situ training for teaching safety skills to children. Educ Treat Child 2009;32(1):63–75.
23. Hardy MS. Teaching firearm safety to children: failure of a program. J Dev Behav Pediatr 2002;23(2):71–6.
24. Hardy MS1, Armstrong FD, Martin BL, et al. A firearm safety program for children: they just can't say no. J Dev Behav Pediatr 1996;17(4):216–21.
25. Jackman GA, Farah MM, Kellermann AL, et al. Seeing is believing: What do boys do when they find a real gun? Pediatrics 2001;107(6):1247–50.
26. Miltenberger RG, Fogel VA, Beck KV, et al. Efficacy of the stranger safety abduction-prevention program and parent-conducted in situ training. J Appl Behav Anal 2013;46(4):817–20.
27. Harriage B, Blair KS, Miltenberger R. An evaluation of a parent implemented in situ pedestrian safety skills intervention for individuals with autism. J Autism Dev Disord 2016;46(6):2017–27.
28. Garcia D, Dukes C, Brady M, et al. Using modeling and rehearsal to teach fire safety to children. J Appl Behav Anal 2016;49:699–704.
29. Miltenberger RG, Gatheridge BJ, Satterlund M, et al. Teaching safety skills to children to prevent gun play: An evaluation of in situ training. J Appl Behav Anal 2005;38(3):395–8.
30. Sanchez S, Miltenberger RG. Evaluating the effectiveness of an abduction prevention program for young adults with intellectual disabilities. Child Fam Behav Ther 2015;37(3):197–207.
31. Carroll LA, Miltenberger R, O'Neill HK. A review and critique of research evaluating child sexual abuse prevention programs. Educ Treat Child 1992;5(4): 335–54.
32. Jostad CM, Miltenberger RG, Kelso P, et al. Peer tutoring to prevent firearm play acquisition, generalization, and long-term maintenance of safety skills. J Appl Behav Anal 2008;41(1):117–23.
33. Ledbetter-Cho K, Lang R, Davenport K, et al. Behavioral skills training to improve the abduction-prevention skills of children with autism. Behav Anal Pract 2016; 9(3):266–70.
34. Page TJ, Iwata BA, Neef NA. Teaching pedestrian skills to retarded persons: generalization from the classroom to the natural environment. J Appl Behav Anal 1976;9(4):433–44.
35. Houvouras IVAJ, Harvey MT. Establishing fire safety skills using behavioral skills training. J Appl Behav Anal 2014;47(2):420–4.
36. Miltenberger RG, Flessner C, Gatheridge B, et al. Evaluation of behavioral skills training to prevent gun play in children. J Appl Behav Anal 2004;37(4):513–6.
37. Tarasenko MA, Miltenberger RG, Brower-Breitwieser C, et al. Evaluation of peer training for teaching abduction prevention skills. Child Fam Behav Ther 2010; 32(3):219–30.
38. Maxfield TC, Miltenberger RG, Novotny MA. Evaluating small-scale simulation for training firearm safety skills. J Appl Behav Anal 2019;52(2):491–8.
39. Neef NA, Iwata BA, Page TJ. Public transportation training: In vivo versus classroom instruction. J Appl Behav Anal 1978;11(3):331–44.
40. Vanselow NR, Hanley GP. An evaluation of computerized behavioral skills training to teach safety skills to young children. J Appl Behav Anal 2014;47:51–69.
41. Çakiroğlu Ü, Gökoğlu S. Development of fire safety behavioral skills via virtual reality. Comput Educ 2019;133:56–68.

Pediatric Prevention
General Prevention

Christopher P. Morley, PhD[a,b,c,*], Alicia C. Reyes, MPH[d]

KEYWORDS

- Prevention • Preventive medicine • Opioids

KEY POINTS

- Prevention may be divided into primary, secondary, and tertiary prevention.
- Prevention can be an abstract concept: it is therefore useful to consider concepts from the medical social sciences when practicing prevention.
- The "Prevention Paradox" describes that although high-risk individuals are more likely to experience a given outcome, most cases come from the broader population.

Then came the fifth and final triumph—the prevention of disease.
—William Osler[1]

The concept of prevention in medicine has a long history, one that likely exceeds that as described by William Osler in 2013. Although the phrase attributed to Benjamin Franklin, that "an ounce of prevention is worth a pound of cure," was describing the prevention of house fires, it is nonetheless often applied to illness as well.

But what do we actually mean when we discuss prevention? A simplistic response might suggest that prevention amounts to stopping a disease from occurring, either through avoidance of risk factors, or through prophylactic measures, such as vaccination, use of barrier methods during sexual encounters, and so forth. However, as one delves into the topic of prevention, it becomes apparent that there are multiple points for intervention into a disease, that the stage of disease matters as to what preventive actions are appropriate, the type of disease (eg, a straightforward, acute condition, such as an infection vs a complex syndrome or chronic condition), and even the overlapping concepts of disease versus illness. Although general definitions of prevention

[a] Department of Public Health and Preventive Medicine, Upstate Medical University, WSK 2262, Syracuse, NY 13210, USA; [b] Department of Family Medicine, Upstate Medical University, WSK 2262, Syracuse, NY 13210, USA; [c] Department of Psychiatry and Behavioral Sciences, Upstate Medical University, WSK 2262, Syracuse, NY 13210, USA; [d] MPH Program Alum, Upstate Medical University, College of Medicine, Syracuse, NY 13210, USA
* Corresponding author. Department of Public Health and Preventive Medicine, Upstate Medical University, WSK 2262, Syracuse, NY 13210.
E-mail address: MorleyCP@upstate.edu
Twitter: @morleycp (C.P.M.)

Pediatr Clin N Am 67 (2020) 585–588
https://doi.org/10.1016/j.pcl.2020.02.012
0031-3955/20/© 2020 Elsevier Inc. All rights reserved.
pediatric.theclinics.com

are readily available to clinicians and health scientists, the purpose of this article was (1) to restate the general framework of primary, secondary, and tertiary prevention; and (2) to describe a lens through which to consider preventive activities. In doing so, we hoped to offer some concepts to keep in mind, as the accompanying topically focused articles in this volume are considered.

PRIMARY, SECONDARY, AND TERTIARY PREVENTION

The standard framework by which to view preventive activities is through primary,[2] secondary,[3] and tertiary[4] prevention. In particular,

- *Primary prevention* describes efforts to stop disease from occurring in individuals who have no history, and no current signs or symptoms, of the disease one is attempting to prevent. Importantly, primary prevention attempts to mitigate the risks of developing a disease before it develops. Examples include vaccination of uninfected individuals, lead abatement in advance of the detection of an elevated blood lead level, the requirement for protective equipment in various activities (eg, helmets, seatbelts), the inspection of food and dining facilities, and so on. In each example given, illness has not yet occurred.
- *Secondary prevention* describes the early identification of disease before it progresses to cause greater morbidity or mortality in an individual. A clear and classic example of secondary prevention is screening for the target condition. Whether screening for autism spectrum disorder (ASD) in very young children, screening for cancer in asymptotic individuals, or screening for domestic abuse, the point in each case is that there is no formal identification of a pathologic process at the time of screening; there may be suspicions that something clinically relevant is occurring (eg, developmental delays, patterns of injury in the case of ASD or domestic abuse, respectively), or there may be no indications that any disease state is present (in the case of asymptomatic or in situ neoplasm).
- *Tertiary prevention* describes effort to mitigate worsening outcomes after a disease process is occurring, or after an acute event has transpired. These efforts could focus on a repeat occurrence of an acute event (eg, prevention of a second cardiovascular event, after a first one has occurred), or they can focus on the prevention of sequalae, occurring downstream from the primary disease. In the latter case, examples include the teaching of life or coping skills for those diagnosed with developmental conditions like ASD, postsurgical infection control, and so forth.

APPLYING PREVENTION IN PRACTICE

Several considerations should come into play when considering theprimary-secondary-tertiary (PST) Prevention framing. Perhaps first, and most obviously, once one is considering where a strategy falls along the prevention continuum, it becomes apparent that disease must be considered along a spectrum of progression, as opposed to a binary "sick/not sick" status. The practical ramification of this point is that there is always something that can be done to prevent progression to a next (and worse) circumstance. In many instances, and often in the case of primary prevention strategies, the individual is (by definition) not sick, and may not be experiencing very severe, or any, precursor signs of impending illness. An individual patient may be experiencing metabolic signs of risk factors for diabetes mellitus or hypertension, for example, but the actual progression to either condition may not truly be "felt" by the patient. When framing how individuals receive preventive measures (either when considering individual-level advice, or population-level policy), the conceptual dichotomy of disease versus illness also may be useful. In an anthropological concept popularized by Kleinman,[5] "disease" in this model refers to the physical manifestation of a malady. This contrasts with illness, which describes the experience of the patient, in naming the illness, feeling the symptoms, and living the ramifications, of having a disease. This dichotomy of a clinically defined disease versus an individually experienced illness may affect prevention efforts, because prevention at any stage seeks to prevent disease (or progression of disease) that the individual has not (yet) experienced as illness. More clearly, risk of a communicable infection in a person with no signs or symptoms is a relatively abstract concept, and abstract concepts tend to be poor motivators to action (such as pursuing vaccination). Perceptions, risk comprehension, and cues to action become vital considerations[6] when convincing patients not just to believe the factual information presented to them in clinic or through public health messaging, but in getting patients and populations to act on the information.

An additional consideration is the importance of the "Prevention Paradox," originally described by Geoffrey Rose and colleagues.[7,8] Although complex in its implications, the core concern expressed in the Prevention Paradox is that cases of disease often arise more frequently in the (larger) pool of low-risk individuals, than in the (smaller) pool of high-risk individuals. That is to say, although high-risk individuals may be at greater likelihood of experiencing a given disease or outcome, most cases come from the broader population. Stemming from this point, one may engage in prevention at the individual or population level.[9] Examples of population-level prevention include universalizing laws about vaccination, helmet or seatbelt usage, or food inspections, as previously described. Individual-level prevention involves direct interaction with, and decision-making by, the patient, and may include lifestyle changes, reduction of salt intake, weight loss, exercise, screening, and so forth.

Although strategies at the 2 levels do not necessarily need to conflict, the paradox comes into play when one wishes to direct population-level preventive interventions toward an entire population, including low-risk individuals. One the one hand, this may be a rather benign issue, as in the case of Naloxone distribution.[10] Naloxone, an opioid agonist, is a first-line response to apparent opioid overdose.[11] Widespread distribution of Naloxone kits is a population strategy designed to prevent death in the case of opioid overdose, but distributing Naloxone widely in a population may result in many low-risk individuals (or individuals at low risk for encountering an overdose, firsthand) carrying Naloxone they will never need or use, to derive some benefit. There is usually little resistance to such a measure, other than from the perspective of resource allocation. On the other hand, widespread vaccination policies create population-level herd immunity, as well as individual benefit. However, regardless of the factual basis (or lack therein), the decision to allow one's child to be vaccinated, or to wear a helmet (or buckle a child into an approved child seat) relies on individual compliance, and assessment of risk. To apply another example, encouraging a patient to quit (or never start) smoking requires the patient to assess his or her own risk of disease or harm, as well as to assess his or her own concerns about the disease at which they are at higher risk by partaking in a particular activity. In other words, individual-level smoking prevention requires the individual to understand the risks of addiction, cancer, heart disease, and other consequences of smoking; apply those risks to oneself; and decide, frankly, if they care more about smoking than about getting sick. However, population-level interventions to combat smoking, including marketing and usage restrictions, as well as economic disincentives (usually through taxes) affect the decision to smoke through changes to the broader population-level context. As such, individual-level prevention may intersect with patient autonomy (or perceptions of autonomy).

Population-level prevention often impacts large numbers of people at low risk for disease to achieve prevention goals.

Taken together, efforts at both the level of the patient and the population to motivate participation in preventive interventions will likely be more successful through the use of careful communication that not only considers the factual basis of the motivation to provide the care, or the assumed authority of the messenger (be it physician, other provider, health care agency, and so forth), but also the perceptions, experiences, and competing messages experienced by the individuals targeted by the intervention, as well as the core abstraction of benefits that patients will likely weigh (either consciously or unconsciously) against their own perceptions of risk, inconvenience, or difficulty. Interventions also will be more successful if they include cultural considerations, and are developed with input from the target community.

ACKNOWLEDGMENTS

The authors are grateful for comments on a draft version of this article provided by Martha Wojtowycz, PhD.

DISCLOSURE

The authors have nothing to disclose.

REFERENCES

1. Osler W. Chapter VI - the rise of preventive medicine. In: The evolution of modern medicine. Project Guttenberg; 2013. Available at: http://www.gutenberg.org/files/1566/1566-h/1566-h.htm#link2HCH0006.
2. Reisig V, Wildner M. Prevention, primary. In: Wilhelm K, editor. Encyclopedia of public health. Dresden: Germany; 2008. p. 1141–3.
3. Wildner M, Nennstiel-Ratzel U. Prevention, secondary. In: Wilhelm K, editor. Encyclopedia of public health. Dresden: Germany; 2008. p. 1141–9.
4. Grill E, Reinhardt JD, Stucki G. Prevention, Tertiary. In: Wilhelm K, editor. Encyclopedia of public health. Dresden: Germany; 2008. p. 1149–51.
5. Kleinman A. The illness narratives: suffering, healing, and the human condition. New York,: Basic Books; 1988.
6. Tubiana S, Launay O, Galtier F, et al. Attitudes, knowledge, and willingness to be vaccinated against seasonal influenza among patients hospitalized with influenza-like-illness: impact of diagnostic testing. Hum Vaccin Immunother 2019. https://doi.org/10.1080/21645515.2019.1674598.
7. Rose GA, Geoffrey A, Khaw K-T, et al. Rose's strategy of preventive medicine: the complete original text. Oxford University Press; 2008.
8. Rose GA. Sick individuals and sick populations. Int J Epidemiol 1985;14(1):32–8.
9. Raza S, Salemi J, Zoorob R. Historical perspectives on prevention paradox: when the population moves as a whole. J Family Med Prim Care 2018;7(6):1163–5.
10. Walley AY, Xuan Z, Hackman HH, et al. Opioid overdose rates and implementation of overdose education and nasal naloxone distribution in Massachusetts: interrupted time series analysis. BMJ 2013;346:f174.
11. Adams J. Surgeon general's advisory on naloxone and opioid overdose. Washington, DC: US Dep Heal Hum Serv; 2018. p. 6–7. Available at: https://www.hhs.gov/surgeongeneral/priorities/opioids-and-addiction/naloxone-advisory/index.html.

Behavior and Substance Addictions in Children
A Behavioral Model and Potential Solutions

Jordan Belisle, PhD[a], Mark R. Dixon, PhD[b],*

KEYWORDS

- Childhood addiction • Behaviorism • Acceptance

KEY POINTS

- Behavior and substance use addictions are increasingly prevalent in children, with increased risk for substance abuse and mental health diagnoses in adulthood.
- The behavioral model emphasizes external context variables, important findings in neuroscience research, as well as how human language and cognition participates in addiction.
- This article proposes a comprehensive model of addiction to inform research on the prevention and treatment of childhood addiction, emphasizing skills training, mindfulness training, and broader treatment strategies consistent with acceptance and commitment therapy.

Children have more access to education and technology today than at any point in human history; yet, rates of behavioral and substance addictions are increasing. According to Gentile and colleagues, an estimated 1% to 9% of children could meet diagnostic criteria for an Internet gaming disorder, with increased risk of depression, poor academic performance, relationship challenges with parents, and higher rates of aggression. In a longitudinal study of twelfth-grade adolescents, Barrington-Trimis and colleagues[1] estimated that smoking increased from 9% in 2004% to 13.7% in 2014, putting children at an elevated risk of smoking in adulthood.[2] According to a recent large-scale analysis of public use files from the National Survey on Drug Use and Health in the United States,[3] 22% of adolescents ages 12 years to 17 years have used alcohol, 12% have used cannabis, 11% have misused prescription medication, and 4% have used other illicit drugs.

What distinguishes the various types of addictions in children is not well defined, and there is debate concerning the inclusion of multiple childhood and adolescent addictions within the *Diagnostic and Statistical Manual of Mental Disorders* (Fifth Edition)

[a] Applied Behavior Analysis, Psychology Department, Missouri State University, 901 S National Avenue, Springfield, MO 65897, USA; [b] Department of Disability and Human Development, University of Illinois at Chicago, Chicago, IL, USA
* Corresponding author. 226 Spring Avenue, Naperville, IL 60540.
E-mail address: mrdixon@uic.edu

Pediatr Clin N Am 67 (2020) 589–602
https://doi.org/10.1016/j.pcl.2020.02.013
0031-3955/20/© 2020 Elsevier Inc. All rights reserved.

(*DSM-V*).[4,5] For example, classifying overeating as a behavioral or substance use disorder can be challenging because, although a food is being consumed, the addictive properties of food may be less direct than other substances (eg, nicotine).

The pragmatic utility of these distinctions also may be limited. Although the *DSM-V* delineates the topography of various addictive behaviors while maintaining construct validity, this approach may lack clinical utility in directing prevention and treatment efforts.[6–8] The *DSM-V* adopts a taxonomic approach to diagnosing mental health disorders that assumes symptoms are evidence for an underlying disorder. As noted by Follette and colleagues,[9,10] such models risk ascribing the cause of disordered symptoms to the disorder itself. This can be seen in how addictions are discussed, such as when a person "has" an addiction that "causes" suffering in some measurable way. The risk is that prevention and treatment are formed around the topography or symptoms of the behavior rather than individualized to address the behavior directly through the underlying motivation that contributes to the maintenance of the behavior.[11]

An alternative conceptualization of addiction is a functional contextual approach that seeks to determine the function (or purpose) of disordered behavior as it occurs within a dynamic context,[12] thus emphasizing the idiosyncratic nature of the behavior. Although the various addictions experienced by children differ in terms of the substance (eg, alcohol) or activity (eg, Internet) consumed, the functional interaction between the disordered behaviors and the context in which they occur may be similar (eg, engaging in addicted behavior produces specific forms of social interaction). Thus, a functional contextual approach may be superior to the taxonomic approach by directing efforts aimed at preventing and treating addiction in children through conceptualization of addiction as an outcome rather than a cause.

There exist several shared symptoms across both behavior and substance addictions,[13,14] such as salience of the addiction in a person's life, euphoria from the activity, tolerance, withdrawal, conflict with other values, and relapse potential. Although the stimulus being consumed may vary, when consumption becomes disordered, seeking the substance becomes a salient part of the child's life at the cost of pursuing other values, and failure to obtain the stimulus can lead to physiologic/psychological withdrawal. According to Alavi and colleagues,[15] there appear to be few differences in the pathology of behavior and substance use addictions. For example, Ko and colleagues[16] demonstrated that neural substrates of cue-elicited urges for gaming in individuals with a gaming addiction resemble cue-elicited craving in other substance use addictions. Furthermore, when access to 1 addictive activity or substance is restricted, individuals with additions may be more likely to transition to other addictive behaviors (eg,.[17–19]) Addiction substitution is problematic in treatment because addictive behavior can become highly resistant and new topographies of behavior might emerge that serve the same function as the original behavior. As noted by Kim and Hodgins,[20] addiction substitution is further evidence that addictive behavior symptoms result from shared underlying mechanisms, requiring a transdiagnostic treatment model with potentially greater utility in prevention and treatment.

Why some children show addictions whereas others do not also must be accounted for. One early predictor of the development of behavior and substance addictions is attention-deficit/hyperactivity disorder (ADHD) (eg, see Ornoy and colleagues,[21] Paulus and colleagues,[22] and Ramano and colleagues[23]) A defining characteristic of ADHD is that attentional processes are at deficit; however, attention to the addictive activity or substance often is salient and pervasive. Lee and Gibbs[24] suggested that adolescents with food addiction demonstrated lower distress tolerance, mirroring the inability of children with ADHD to attend to potentially distressing activities (eg, schoolwork). Roos and colleagues[25] and others[26,27] have suggested that early life stressors can compromise the development of affective neural networks that increase responsiveness to negative or threatening stimuli and participate in emotional recognition and other social behaviors, implicating low social competence as a strong predictor of addictive behavior. Carliner and colleagues[28] also have documented that exposure to potentially traumatic events prior to age 11 places children at greater risk for addictive behavior (see also Moustafa and colleagues[29]).

A functional approach to conceptualizing addiction may be possible by examining these processes in the service of developing preventative and treatment procedures. Xu and colleagues evaluated motivational factors that may predict online gaming addictions among adolescents. It seems intuitive that rewards embedded within games (eg, points and progressing in the game) could serve to strengthen addictive gaming behavior, yet Xu and colleagues found that only the need for escape from stress and seeking of peer relationships were predictive of disordered levels of gaming. These motivational factors may become exacerbated for children who already demonstrate diminished affective responding resulting in lowered stress tolerance and lower social competence. This result closely resembles research on gambling addictions in adults, showing that although gambling can be maintained by several idiosyncratic functions, disordered gambling is disproportionately maintained by escape from negative social or relationship functions.[30] Thus, some addictive behavior may be conceptualized as motivated by escape, access to rewards, access to social interactions, and underlying physiologic variables.[31]

In the sections that follow, the authors contend that by defining addiction in terms of the dynamic interaction between addictive behavior and the context in which it occurs, rather than by its topography, solutions may be forthcoming that directly address factors that influence addictions in children. Some potential solutions are discussed for the prevention and treatment of addictions in children that are consistent with a functional contextual approach, including acceptance and commitment therapy (ACT) (see Hayes and colleagues[32]) that has been put forward as a transdiagnostic intervention for several disorders classified within the *DSM-V*.[33–36]

FACTORS INFLUENCING ADDICTIVE BEHAVIOR IN CHILDREN
Tangible Rewards

Behavioral models of addiction emphasize tangible rewards, which, in the context of addictive behavior in children, can take the form of points accessed in a game or toys that often are paired with unhealthy fast food options. According to King and colleagues,[37] parallels can be drawn between gambling and the structural characteristics of video gaming, which allow the user to control various aspects of a game, and points or credits are awarded probabilistically based on performance. Developers delineate the manipulation of video game rewards to encourage prolonged play into social features, manipulation and control features, reward and punishment features, and reward presentation features, all of which have been shown to have an impact on patterns on gaming in children.[38] Toys embedded in unhealthy food options also may promote consumption of unhealthy foods. For example, Hobin and colleagues[39] presented children with healthier and unhealthy versions of McDonald's Happy Meals. When a toy was obtainable only as part of the healthier option, children were likely to forego the unhealthy option; unfortunately, toys often are paired with unhealthy foods, potentially establishing a preference for high-calorie food over time.

Access to peer interaction also may contribute to addictive behavior. Food, gaming, and drug use provide a potential social activity allowing for exchanges with others that are centered around the addictive activity. For example, when gaming online, many children concurrently converse with other gamers. Given that social skill deficits are a predictor of childhood addictions,[26,27] they may function to increase risk by enhancing the value of social interaction with similar peers for at least 2 reasons. First, limited social skills may result in deprivation of positive social interactions with peers, increasing the overall value of all social interactions, including maladaptive social behavior like excessive gaming or drug use. Second, because children with addictions are engaging in a joint task, deficits may be less pronounced in that context because members of the social group can discuss the object of joint attention (eg, discussing the game).

Physiologic Rewards

Physiologic mechanisms also are implicated in addictive behavior, as evidenced within the high and euphoria experienced through consumption of addictive substances and, in some cases, access to peer interactions. Dopaminergic pathways are particularly implicated,[40–44] and some addiction can be understood as the concurrent action of multiple neural networks that, when activated, lead to overt addictive behavior. For example, when a child picks up a game controller, cigarette, or illicit substance, specific neural pathways are activated. Dopamine release strengthens the neural pathways that preceded the activity, increasing the probability that the same neural pathways activate under similar contextual conditions. Therefore, the chain of behaviors that contribute to addictive behavior (eg, purchasing, preparing, and consuming a drug) become linked in a reward system. Because addictive substances directly stimulate the reward pathway, this is considered automatic sources of reinforcement (**Fig. 1**).

Escape/Avoidance Mechanisms

Although tangible rewards and physiologic mechanisms undoubtedly influence addictive behavior, these rewards only partly predict addictive behavior. Perhaps to an even greater extent, escape from stress or avoidance can have a considerable impact on addictive behavior. Examples include escape from life stressors and escape from thoughts that contribute to addiction in the lives of children. Engaging in behavior that removes or attenuates an aversive context is one of the greatest predictors of gaming addiction and smoking in children and adolescents.[45–47] Snodgrass and

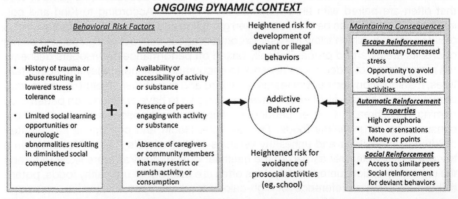

Fig. 1. A functional contextual model of external environmental factors that may increase risk and maintain addictive behavior in children.

colleagues[48] found that video game players were more likely to engage in excessive play when experiencing elevated life stress. These data further support that gaming can provide a cognitive diversion from stressful thoughts that co-occur with life stress. Similarly, nicotine also can serve to momentarily relieve stress, because is a common reason for smoking reported by adult smokers.[49,50] Hajek and colleagues[51] provided data from an adult smoking treatment program showing that smoking cessation led to lowered levels of stress longer term, supporting the potential for an escape function in the context of smoking. In sum, multiple processes are expressed as contributing factors to addictions in children (see **Fig. 1**).

Contextual Factors

Antecedent contextual factors are events that precede addictive behavior and may make the addictive behavior more likely (see **Fig. 1**). Availability of the activity or substance can make use more likely. For example, if a child does not have immediate access to video games, use may be less likely in the moment. Although this seems intuitive, modeled in this way, environmental modifications can be forthcoming to reduce addictive behavior, at least in the short term (eg, restricting access to games). Likewise, access to others who engage in addictive behavior may play a role in addictive behavior for some activities. Bahr and colleagues,[52] Barnes-Holmes and colleagues,[53] and Barrington-Trimis and colleagues[54] sampled 4230 adolescents and found that peer drug use was a direct predictor of drug use in children, with parent/sibling drug use as a predictor that may interact indirectly with peer use further elevating the risk of substance abuse. Parent monitoring of children was a significant but small predictor of adolescent substance abuse.

Delay Discounting

Delay discounting describes a preference for smaller immediate rewards over larger delayed rewards, even when this leads to a reduction in amount of obtained reinforcement over time.[55] That is, the subjective value of a reinforcer diminishes as a function of time (delay) to receiving that reinforcement. Delay discounting often is described as a model of impulsive behavior and may be a fundamental behavioral process underlying addictive behavior.[56] As evidence, in a recent meta-analysis,[57,58] the relationship between delay discounting and addictive behavior in adults was robust, and this is consistent across different topographies of addictive behavior and across several different measures of delay discounting. Thus, delay discounting may explain why children gravitate toward the smaller immediate reinforcers available through gaming, excessive food consumption, or use of illicit substances, rather than larger delayed reinforcers that otherwise may be available in absence of the addictive behavior.

Psychological Functions

Any model of addictive behavior in children should recognize the role of language and cognitive capabilities.[59,60] Relational frame theory (RFT)[61] is an account of human cognitive and language development that is relevant to the present analysis. Broadly speaking, within RFT, a relation between stimuli emerges in the absence of direct pairing. **Fig. 2** provides an example of this type of relation in the context of addictive behavior. Using cigarette use as the example, A is the context in which cigarette use occurs and B is the actual cigarette itself. The A = B relation can be established through temporal contiguity, where the context occurs immediately prior to and concurrently with the cigarette. Thus, seeing the cigarette is associated with the context (B = A). The context (A) also may be related to a word describing the context

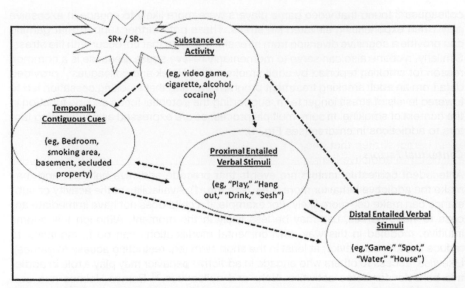

Fig. 2. Exemplar model of entailed verbal relations participating in addictive behavior. SR+/SR- represent directly experienced positive and negative reinforcement contingencies, respectively. Solid arrows represent directly paired relations. Dashed arrows represent derived relations. Proximal entailed stimuli are those more closely related to SR+/SR- functions and distal entailed stimuli are those less closely related to SR+/SR- functions.

(B) (A = C). For example, if the phrase, "hang out," comes to refer to the location where cigarettes are smoked, then the phrase, "hang out," is related to the context (C = A). Consequently, through the shared relation associated with smoking, the phrase, "hang out," can be related to a cigarette even in the absence of a location (C = B). This relation may be actualized when, for example, the phrase, "hang out," applies to a new context that results in smoking.

Given such pairings, words may come to evoke addictive behavior. As shown in **Fig. 2**, the cigarette carries the functions described previously. It produces reinforcement through dopaminergic activation, social interaction, and escape from stressors as well as escape from withdrawals. In this framework, these functions can transfer across stimuli. For example, when a person is in the context (A) w,here smoking occurs even if friends are not present or a cigarette is not accessible, physiologic changes may begin consistent with preparation for cigarette consumption (ie, cue reactivity). The cue for smoking elicits physiologic responses consistent with use of the drug, whereas failure to obtain the drug can result in even greater sensations of withdrawal. Likewise, words related to the drug (eg, smoke and cigarette) or the context (eg, hang out) also obtain similar functions, such that these words alone can lead to physiologic preparatory responses. Likewise, nonrelated words also may obtain the functions maintaining use of the drug (see **Fig. 2**). For example, even though "spot" is not directly associated with smoking or cigarettes, its pairing with the phrase "hang out" could result in the transfer of function, such that the word "spot" evokes the behavior.

In contrast to RFT, relational density theory (RDT)[62] provides a further conceptual model to include the impact of resistance to external influences over the contextual cues associated with a given behavior. For example, small prosmoking biases in adolescence are predictive of smoking behavior[63,64]; however, as the smoker contacts preferred experiences around (eg, interactions with peers, increases in dopamine, and escape from stress), the bias may be strengthened and, therefore, may become more resistant to change.

The evolution of relations among cues may be problematic, especially in the context of children and adolescents demonstrating addictive behavior. Belisle and Dixon (in press)[65] (Belisle, J, Clayton, M. Coherence and the Merging of Relational Classes in Self-Organizing Networks: Extending Relational Density Theory, submitted for publication). Relational gravity: Predicting the merging of equivalence classes through pre-experimental relational coherence. *Journal of Contextual Behavior Science*) demonstrated that because there were more relational cues associated with an analog to addictive behavior, participants were more likely to acquire new relations without direct teaching. One common symptom reported by individuals with addictions is the salience or pervasiveness of thoughts surrounding the addictive activity or substance. That is, several stimuli within the environment, including novel stimuli never before associated with the activity or substance, have the potential to evoke cues contained within the addictive class. RDT may explain this outcome in that, as the number of addictive cues, the probability that new stimuli will obtain addictive functions strengthens even further. The totality of this model is provided in **Fig. 3**.

AVENUES FOR PREVENTION AND TREATMENT OF ADDICTIONS IN CHILDREN

The authors' model, described throughout this article, can provide several avenues for treatment, because, ultimately, the validity of any conceptual model must come from its success in informing effective interventions.[66] In visiting potential prevention and treatment strategies, the authors focus on risk factors, diminished social skills, levels of dopaminergic activity, a history of trauma, delay discounting, and organizing relations among contextual cues.

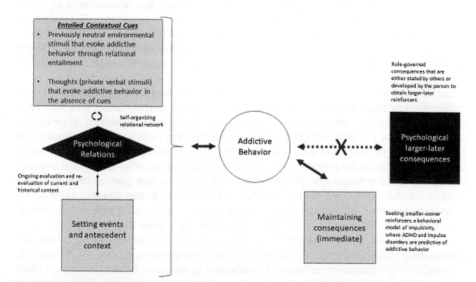

Fig. 3. A functional contextual model of psychological or relational factors that may increase risk and maintain addictive behavior in children. "smaller sooner" refers to smaller more immediate positive and negative reinforcers, and "larger later" refers to larger and more delayed abstracted reinforcers.

With regard to diminished social skills, behavioral skills training has been shown efficacious in teaching adaptive social skills across clinical populations (eg, see Baton and colleagues,[67] Belisle,[68] Ryan and colleagues,[69] and Smith and colleagues[70]) and to result in higher rates of social interaction in the natural environment (eg, see Stewart and colleauges[71]). Such an approach also may offset those social contingencies that maintain addictive behavior because opportunities by making opportunities for social interaction not centered around an addictive activity or substance more immediately available for children.

Prevention efforts also should focus on limiting children's exposure to trauma or violence, and, when trauma or violence does occur, to intentionally target stress tolerance as a preventative behavioral process in children. This is an area that requires considerably greater research, but some inferences can be made from stress research with other populations. For example, Welle and Graf[72] and Wilson and colleagues[73] identified factors that may be associated with higher stress tolerance in college students, primarily avoidance of addictive substances. The authors highlighted the importance of coping skills, which provide readily identifiable behaviors that can be taught for children. One such strategy may be promoting mindful behaviors in children. Mindfulness-based stress reduction strategies are supported with children in the reduction of stress-related hormones, reported stress, and social anxiety,[74–76] all of which appear to contribute specifically to addictive behavior.

Vidrine and colleagues[77] compared a mindfulness-based addiction treatment to traditional cognitive behavior therapy for adult smokers, supporting mindfulness-based treatments as potentially more effective. Neurologic models supporting the effectiveness of mindfulness-based strategies on the treatment of addiction also are emerging, supporting a relationship between mindfulness and the stress-reducing escape functions of substance abuse.[78–80] Wilson and colleagues[81] cautioned that there are several potential barriers to implementation of this technology that must be further researched and addressed, and greater research also is needed to develop mindfulness strategies developed specifically for children and adolescents to target addictions at initial conditions; however, this research is emerging. For example, Yoo and colleagues[82] evaluated the efficacy of a school-based mindfulness program for children on rates of cellphone addiction. Results supported not only a reduction in cellphone use after mindfulness intervention but also reduction in depression and anxiety symptoms.

Social skills training and mindfulness-based strategies directly address the social contingencies associated with addictive behavior but may not readily address delay discounting of larger delayed rewards associated with nonuse. Research on delay discounting across the lifespan conducted by Göllner and colleagues[83] suggests that future episodic thinking and goal-oriented behavior were predictive of a greater ability to delay gratification for children and adults, providing a potential behavioral process to target directly in treatment. In the authors' model, addictive behaviors provide access to smaller immediate reinforcers at the expense of larger delayed reinforcers. Strategies could be developed to redirect attention to delayed goals in the context where addictive behavior is most likely. For example, rather than punishing a child for engaging in excessive video gaming, some success may be achieved by redirecting the child toward delayed reinforcers like performing well in school. Bromberg and colleagues[84] evaluated the efficacy of redirecting to episodic future thinking on rates of delay discounting in adolescents, showing a significant reduction in delay discounting rates relative to control trials where redirection did not occur.

These strategies and others are contained within ACT as a broader approach to behavioral and psychological treatment. ACT targets psychological flexibility, or the persistence or adaptation of behavior to maximize contact with values-based contingencies while willingly contacting private and public stimuli in the present environment.[85] Psychological flexibility is achieved through strengthening of at-least 6 core processes. Values and committed action include redirection to future-oriented thinking but focusing on core values and measurable actions that can lead a person closer to those values. For example, if an adolescent with an addiction values family, committed actions are behaviors that the adolescent can engage in that move closer to this identified value. Present moment awareness can include mindfulness training to increase a person's contact with public and private stimuli that occur. In the context of addictive behavior, present moment awareness and acceptance processes necessarily must co-occur, because stress associated with nonuse as well as the saliency of the addiction occurs in the present moment and requires momentary acceptance of aversive experience, again in the service of moving closer to identified values and to engage in committed action. Cognitive defusion and self-as-context directly address the self-organizing relations and behaviors associated with addictive behavior by several studies support the use of ACT-based strategies in the treatment of addictive behavior in adults, including smoking,[86] substance abuse (see Lee and colleauges[87] for initial meta-analysis), and pornography.[88]

Additional research is needed to evaluate the effectiveness of ACT as a treatment model for children experiencing addiction. ACT is increasingly adapted for use with children to address several behaviors. Swain and colleagues[89] conducted a systematic review of research evaluating ACT with children experiencing a variety of mental health and behavioral challenges and included 21 studies with more than 700 research participants. Results supported the use of ACT strategies in reducing anxiety and depression with children as well as overall increases in quality-of-life measures. Although additional research is needed, one potential technology involves ACT-based protocols that can be implemented at a school-wide level to combat growing rates of addictive behavior in children. For example, Accept. Identify. Move. (AIM)[90] is a curriculum that contains ACT-based strategies with an emphasis on mindfulness training and direct contingency management strategies. By addressing behavioral environmental factors and psychological verbal relations concurrently, AIM or similar technologies could be exceptionally advantageous in preventing and treating addictive behavior. The manualization of AIM allows for evaluations through conventional testing methods, such as single-case experimental designs and randomized control trials, and the authors encourage researchers to begin to evaluate this and similar technologies empirically.

DISCLOSURE

The authors have nothing to disclose.

REFERENCES

1. Barrington-Trimis JL, Urman R, Leventhal AM, et al. E-cigarettes, cigarettes, and the prevalence of adolescent tobacco use. Pediatrics 2016;138:e20153983.
2. Leventhal AM, Stone MD, Andrabi N, et al. Association of e-cigarette vaping and progression to heavier patterns of cigarette smoking. JAMA 2016;316:1918–20.
3. Carmona J, Maxwell JC, Park JY, et al. Prevalence and health characteristics of prescription opioid use, misuse, and use disorders among US adolescents. J Adolesc Health 2020. https://doi.org/10.1016/j.jadohealth.2019.11.306.
4. Gentile DA, Bailey K, Bavelier D, et al. Internet gaming disorder in children and adolescents. Pediatrics 2017;140:S81–5.

5. Kardefelt-Winther D, Heeren A, Schimmenti A, et al. How can we conceptualize behavioural addiction without pathologizing common behaviours? Addiction 2017;112:1709–15.
6. Mullins-Sweatt SN, Widiger TA. Clinical utility and DSM-V. Psychol Assess 2009; 21:302.
7. Mundkur N. Neuroplasticity in children. Indian J Pediatr 2005;72:855–7.
8. Nastally BL, Dixon MR, Jackson JW. Manipulating slot machine preference in problem gamblers through contextual control. J Appl Behav Anal 2010;43:125–9.
9. Follette WC, Bach PA, Follette VM. A behavior-analytic view of psychological health. Behav Anal 1993;16:303–16.
10. Follette WC, Houts AC, Hayes SC. Behavior therapy and the new medical model. Behav Assess 1992;14:323.
11. Eifert GH. More theory-driven and less diagnosis-based behavior therapy. J Behav Ther Exp Psychiatry 1996;27:75–86.
12. Vilardaga R, Hayes SC, Levin ME, et al. Creating a strategy for progress: a contextual behavioral science approach. Behav Anal 2009;32:105–33.
13. Brown RIF. Some contributions of the study of gambling to the study of other addictions. In: Eadington WR, Cornelius JA, editors. Gambling behavior and problem gambling. Reno (Nevada): University of Nevada; 1993. p. 241–72.
14. Kuss DJ, Griffiths MD. Online gaming addiction in children and adolescents: A review of empirical research. J Behav Addict 2012. https://doi.org/10.1556/JBA.1.2012.1.1.
15. Alavi SS, Ferdosi M, Jannatifard F, et al. Behavioral addiction versus substance addiction: correspondence of psychiatric and psychological views. Int J Prev Med 2012;3:290–4.
16. Ko CH, Liu GC, Hsiao S, et al. Brain activities associated with gaming urge of online gaming addiction. J Psychiatr Res 2009;43:739–47.
17. Blanco C, Potenza MN, Kim SW, et al. A pilot study of impulsivity and compulsivity in pathological gambling. Psychiatry Res 2009;167:161–8.
18. Hodgins DC, Kim HS, Stea JN. Increase and decrease of other substance use during recovery from cannabis use disorders. Psychol Addict Behav 2017;31: 727–34.
19. Holliday ED, Logue SF, Oliver C, et al. Stress and nicotine during adolescence disrupts adult hippocampal-dependent learning and alters stress reactivity. Addict Biol 2019;e12769. https://doi.org/10.1111/adb.12769.
20. Kim HS, Hodgins DC. Component model of addiction treatment: a pragmatic transdiagnostic treatment model of behavioral and substance addictions. Front Psychiatry 2018;9:1–17.
21. Ornoy A, Finkel-Pekarsky V, Peles E, et al. ADHD risk alleles associated with opiate addiction: study of addicted parents and their children. Pediatr Res 2016;80:228–36.
22. Paulus FW, Sinzig J, Mayer H, et al. Computer gaming disorder and ADHD in young children—a population-based study. Int J Ment Health Addict 2018;16: 1193–207.
23. Romano M, Truzoli R, Osborne LA, et al. The relationship between autism quotient, anxiety, and internet addiction. Res Autism Spectr Disord 2014;8:1521–6.
24. Lee A, Gibbs SE. Neurobiology of food addiction and adolescent obesity prevention in low-and middle-income countries. J Adolesc Health 2013;52:S39–42.
25. Roos LE, Horn S, Berkman ET, et al. Leveraging translational neuroscience to inform early intervention and addiction prevention for children exposed to early life stress. Neurobiol Stress 2018;9:231–40.

26. Gentile DA, Choo H, Liau A, et al. Pathological video game use among youths: a two-year longitudinal study. Pediatrics 2011;127:e319–29.

27. Lemmens JS, Valkenburg PM, Peter J. Psychosocial causes and consequences of pathological gaming. Comput Hum Behav 2011;27:144–52.

28. Carliner H, Keyes KM, McLaughlin KA, et al. Childhood trauma and illicit drug use in adolescence: a population-based national comorbidity survey replication–adolescent supplement study. J Am Acad Child Adolesc Psychiatry 2016;55:701–8.

29. Moustafa AA, Parkes D, Fitzgerald L, et al. The relationship between childhood trauma, early-life stress, and alcohol and drug use, abuse, and addiction: an integrative review. Curr Psychol 2018. https://doi.org/10.1007/s12144-018-9973-9.

30. Dixon MR, Whiting SW, Gunnarsson KF, et al. Trends in behavior-analytic gambling research and treatment. Behav Anal 2015;38:179–202.

31. Dixon MR, Wilson AN, Belisle J, et al. A functional analytic approach to understanding disordered gambling. Psychol Rec 2018;68:177–87.

32. Hayes SC, Luoma JB, Bond FW, et al. Acceptance and commitment therapy: model, processes and outcomes. Behav Res Ther 2006;44:1–25.

33. Dindo L, Van Liew JR, Arch JJ. Acceptance and commitment therapy: a transdiagnostic behavioral intervention for mental health and medical conditions. Neurotherapeutics 2017;14:546–53.

34. Dixon MR, Holton B. Altering the magnitude of delay discounting by pathological gamblers. J Appl Behav Anal 2009;42:269–75.

35. Dixon MR, Jacobs EA, Sanders S. Contextual control of delay discounting by pathological gamblers. J Appl Behav Anal 2006;39:413–22.

36. Hayes SC, Pistorello J, Levin ME. Acceptance and commitment therapy as a unified model of behavior change. Couns Psychol 2012;40:976–1002.

37. King D, Delfabbro P, Griffiths M. Video game structural characteristics: A new psychological taxonomy. Int J Ment Health Addict 2010;8:90–106.

38. McBride J, Derevensky J. Gambling and video game playing among youth. Journal of Gambling 2017;34:156–78.

39. Hobin EP, Hammond DG, Daniel S, et al. The Happy Meal® effect: the impact of toy premiums on healthy eating among children in Ontario, Canada. Can J Public Health 2012;103:e244–8.

40. Blum K, Chen AL, Giordano J, et al. The addictive brain: all roads lead to dopamine. J Psychoactive Drugs 2012;44:134–43.

41. Blum K, Thanos PK, Oscar-Berman M, et al. Dopamine in the brain: hypothesizing surfeit or deficit links to reward and addiction. J Reward Defic Syndr 2015;1: 95–104.

42. Bricker JB, Mull KE, Kientz JA, et al. Randomized, controlled pilot trial of a smartphone app for smoking cessation using acceptance and commitment therapy. Drug Alcohol Depend 2014;143:87–94.

43. Davis C, Levitan RD, Kaplan AS, et al. Reward sensitivity and the D2 dopamine receptor gene: A case-control study of binge eating disorder. Prog Neuropsychopharmacol Biol Psychiatry 2008;32:620–8.

44. Dias TGC, Wilson VB, Bathula DR, et al. Reward circuit connectivity relates to delay discounting in children with attention-deficit/hyperactivity disorder. Eur Neuropsychopharmacol 2013;23:33–45.

45. Juon HS, Shin Y, Nam JJ. Cigarette smoking among Korean adolescents: prevalence and correlates. Adolescence 1995;30:631–43.

46. Kassel JD, Stroud LR, Paronis CA. Smoking, stress, and negative affect: correlation, causation, and context across stages of smoking. Psychol Bull 2003;129:270–304.
47. Xu Z, Turel O, Yuan Y. Online game addiction among adolescents: motivation and prevention factors. Eur J Inf Syst 2012;21:321–40.
48. Snodgrass JG, Lacy MG, Dengah HF II, et al. A vacation from your mind: Problematic online gaming is a stress response. Comput Hum Behav 2014;38:248–60.
49. Dani JA, Harris RA. Nicotine addiction and comorbidity with alcohol abuse and mental illness. Nat Neurosci 2005;8:1465–70.
50. Todd M. Daily processes in stress and smoking: effects of negative events, nicotine dependence, and gender. Psychol Addict Behav 2004;18:31–9.
51. Hajek P, Taylor T, McRobbie H. The effect of stopping smoking on perceived stress levels. Addiction 2010;105:1466–71.
52. Bahr SJ, Hoffmann JP, Yang X. Parental and peer influences on the risk of adolescent drug use. J Prim Prev 2005;26:529–51.
53. Barnes-Holmes D, Barnes-Holmes Y, Stewart I, et al. A sketch of the implicit relational assessment procedure (IRAP) and the relational elaboration and coherence (REC) model. Psychol Rec 2010;60:527–42.
54. Barrington-Trimis JL, Berhane K, Unger JB, et al. The e-cigarette social environment, e-cigarette use, and susceptibility to cigarette smoking. J Adolesc Health 2016;59:75–80.
55. Odum AL. Delay discounting: I'm a k, you're a k. J Exp Anal Behav 2011;96:427–39.
56. Bickel WK, Johnson MW. Delay discounting: a fundamental behavioral process of drug dependence. In: Loewenstein G, Read D, Baumeister R, editors. Time and decision: economic and psychological perspectives on intertemporal choice. New York: Russell Sage Foundation; 2003. p. 419–40.
57. Amlung M, Vedelago L, Acker J, et al. Steep delay discounting and addictive behavior: a meta-analysis of continuous associations. Addiction 2017;112:51–62.
58. Baer DM, Wolf MM, Risley TR. Some current dimensions of applied behavior analysis 1. J Appl Behav Anal 1968;1:91–7.
59. Dymond S, Roche B, Barnes-Holmes D. The continuity strategy, human behavior, and behavior analysis. Psychol Rec 2003;53:333–47.
60. Hughes S, Barnes-Holmes D. Associative concept learning, stimulus equivalence, and relational frame theory: Working out the similarities and differences between human and non-human behavior. J Exp Anal Behav 2014;101:156–60.
61. Hayes SC, Barnes-Holmes D, Roche B, editors. Relational frame theory: a post-skinnerian account of human language and cognition. New York: Plenum Press; 2001.
62. Belisle J, Dixon MR. Relational density theory: Non-linearity of equivalence relating examined through higher-order volumetric-mass-density. Perspect Behav Sci 2020.
63. Cagney S, Harte C, Barnes-Holmes D, et al. Response biases on the IRAP for adults and adolescents with respect to smokers and nonsmokers: The impact of parental smoking status. Psychol Rec 2017;67:473–83.
64. Critchfield TS. Translational contributions of the experimental analysis of behavior. Behav Anal 2011;34:3–17.
65. Belisle J, Dixon MR. An exploratory analysis of relational density theory: Relational resistance and gravity. Journal of Contextual Behavior Science, in press.
66. Moore J. Behavior analytic pragmatism. J Mind Behav 2016;37:219–45.

67. Baton E, Crosland K, Haynes R. An evaluation of a social skills application for children who are homeless. Res Soc Work Pract 2019;29:323–32.
68. Belisle J. Model dependent realism in a pragmatic science of human behavior. Perspect Behav Sci 2020;16:80–95.
69. Ryan G, Brady S, Holloway J, et al. Increasing appropriate conversation skills using a behavioral skills training package for adults with intellectual disability and autism spectrum disorder. J Intellect Disabil 2019;23:567–80.
70. Smith TE, Bellack AS, Liberman RP. Social skills training for schizophrenia: Review and future directions. Clin Psychol Rev 1996;16:599–617.
71. Stewart KK, Carr JE, LeBlanc LA. Evaluation of family-implemented behavioral skills training for teaching social skills to a child with Asperger's disorder. Clin Case Stud 2007;6:252–62.
72. Welle PD, Graf HM. Effective lifestyle habits and coping strategies for stress tolerance among college students. Am J Health Educ 2011;42:96–105.
73. Wilson VB, Mitchell SH, Musser ED, et al. Delay discounting of reward in ADHD: application in young children. J Child Psychol Psychiatry 2011;52:256–64.
74. Greenberg MT, Harris AR. Nurturing mindfulness in children and youth: current state of research. Child Dev Perspect 2012;6:161–6.
75. Zenner C, Herrnleben-Kurz S, Walach H. Mindfulness-based interventions in schools—a systematic review and meta-analysis. Front Psychol 2014;5:603–20.
76. Zlomke KR, Dixon MR. Modification of slot-machine preferences through the use of a conditional discrimination paradigm. J Appl Behav Anal 2006;39:351–61.
77. Vidrine JI, Spears CA, Heppner WL, et al. Efficacy of mindfulness-based addiction treatment (MBAT) for smoking cessation and lapse recovery: A randomized clinical trial. J Consult Clin Psychol 2016;84:824–38.
78. Garland E. Restructuring reward processing with mindfulness-oriented recovery enhancement: novel therapeutic mechanisms to remediate hedonic dysregulation in addiction, stress, and pain. Ann N Y Acad Sci 2016;1373:25–37.
79. Garland E, Froeliger B, Howard M. Mindfulness training targets neurocognitive mechanisms of addiction at the attention-appraisal-emotion interface. Front Psychiatry 2014;4:173–84.
80. Gentile D. Pathological video-game use among youth ages 8 to 18: a national study. Psychol Sci 2009;20:594–602.
81. Wilson AD, Roos CR, Robinson CS, et al. Mindfulness-based interventions for addictive behaviors: Implementation issues on the road ahead. Psychol Addict Behav 2017;31:888–96.
82. Yoo YG, Lee MJ, Yu B, et al. The effect of mind subtraction meditation on smartphone addiction in school children. Glob J Health Sci 2019;11:16–28.
83. Göllner LM, Ballhausen N, Kliegel M, et al. Delay of gratification, delay discounting and their associations with age, episodic future thinking, and future time perspective. Front Psychol 2018;8:2304–24.
84. Bromberg U, Lobatcheva M, Peters J. Episodic future thinking reduces temporal discounting in healthy adolescents. PLoS One 2017;12:e0188079.
85. Bond FW, Hayes SC, Barnes-Holmes D. Psychological flexibility, ACT, and organizational behavior. Journal of Organizational Behavior Management 2006;26(1-2):25–54.
86. Hernández-López M, Luciano MC, Bricker JB, et al. Acceptance and commitment therapy for smoking cessation: a preliminary study of its effectiveness in comparison with cognitive behavioral therapy. Psychol Addict Behav 2009;23:723–30.

87. Lee EB, An W, Levin ME, et al. An initial meta-analysis of Acceptance and Commitment Therapy for treating substance use disorders. Drug Alcohol Depend 2015;155:1–7.

88. Twohig MP, Crosby JM. Acceptance and commitment therapy as a treatment for problematic internet pornography viewing. Behav Ther 2010;41:285–95.

89. Swain J, Hancock K, Dixon A, et al. Acceptance and commitment therapy for children: a systematic review of intervention studies. J Contextual Behav Sci 2015; 4(2):73–85.

90. Dixon MR, Paliliunas D. Accept. Identify. Move. Carbondale (IL): Shawnee Scientific Press; 2018.

Printed and bound by CPI Group (UK) Ltd, Croydon, CR0 4YY

03/10/2024

01040403-0012